Current Approaches

Obesity

Edited by
W P T James & S W Parker

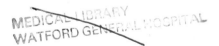

duphar
medical relations

First published 1988

ISBN 1-870678-07-9

Printed in Great Britain by
Inprint (Litho) Ltd., Southampton.

CONTENTS

Editor's Foreword

This book reflects the views of a number of specialists who have spent many years working out how best to assess obesity and how to make treatment most effective. The early chapters set out some of the new views on the interactions between diet and the constitutive tendency to obesity and how this may relate to the other metabolic abnormalities.

Dr. Marks puts forward an intriguing view of how high fat diets might mediate their effects in the susceptible individual by producing an exaggerated response in gastric inhibitory peptide and there is then a series of articles on different aspects of management. The search for new thermogenic drugs as distinct from anorectic agents is certainly an emerging phenomenon, but with so much experience of anorectic drugs one must necessarily be cautious about their acceptability, particularly as it is increasingly recognised that it is the longterm management of obesity which is of fundamental importance to the health of the patient.

Very low calorie diets are dealt with only briefly in the discussion but this is certainly an increasingly popular therapy with new formulations providing much greater reassurance of safety than the earlier nutritionally inadequate formulations being produced, particularly in the United States. As patients struggle to conform to the dietary suggestions of physicians, dietitians and commercial group leaders, they are assailed by a number of physiological and psychological problems which Professor Crisp has brought out very elegantly in his chapter.

One cannot claim that this book highlights a major advance in our understanding of the management of obesity, but it does describe the steady evolution of knowledge and the improvement in our ability to help patients who hitherto have been much neglected by the medical profession.

WPT James
Director
Rowett Research Institute
Aberdeen

iv

CURRENT STATUS OF RESEARCH:
WHY DO PEOPLE GET FAT?

M E J Lean
Consultant Physician
Aberdeen Royal Infirmary

INTRODUCTION
The Weight of the Problem

To the question "Why do people get fat" there are two broad answers possible: either through gluttony and sloth, or through a metabolic disposition (whose expression might nevertheless require some degree of environmental or behavioural input). That overweight is viewed as a major problem is probably self-evident, but should it actually be considered as a disease? The sheer size of the problem can be assessed from the annual expenditures on various efforts to lose weight (Figure 1), together with the combined circulations of the top six slimming magazines of 800,000 with sales of about £5,000,000 per annum, all of which says a great deal about the perceived need for weight loss in the community and for the power of modern promotion of slimming products. Paradoxically, the continued increase in the slimming food market strongly suggests that people are not getting thin and achieving long term success since this should take them out of the market.

The medical consequences of obesity, with its contribution to premature death and chronic illness from a variety of conditions are undisputed, but it is hard to measure their overall costs. In 1981 the costs to the NHS of obesity *per se* were estimated at £14,000,000 and the contribution of obesity to the NHS through the complication of maturity onset diabetes at £67,000,000 (Laing, 1981). It also contributes significantly to the bills for respiratory, cardiovascular and biliary tract diseases, certain cancers and non-specifically to most forms of surgery and to the long term care of the elderly. On top of all this there is a collossal unmeasurable cost in terms of human suffering.

In what sense, though, is obesity *per se* a disease? Many people like being fat. Barbara Wooton once defined pathology as anything the state spends money to prevent. In that sense, it begins to be questionable whether obesity would qualify. The NHS currently spends about £5,000,000 per annum in its efforts to combat obesity - mainly by providing dietitians, who spend 20% of their time on obesity, plus an annual bill for anti-obesity drugs of perhaps £1, 500,000. It is hard to imagine that Barbara Wooton's cirterion would be met by the tiny proportion of this rather small sum which is directed towards prevention. The managers of the NHS might well focus more clearly on combatting obesity after a full analysis of its costs, but then only if treatment can be shown to be effective. Even the most committed

1

dietitian might have difficulty in balancing a cost-benefit analysis of her unequal struggle in the obesity clinic, and few of us would be prepared to stake our careers on the current medical management of obesity.

Figure 1: ANNUAL SIZE OF UK SLIMMING AIDS AND FOODS MARKET
Source: Mintel Publications

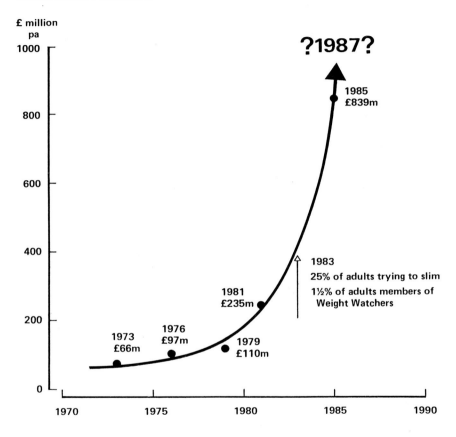

Before effective treatment can be developed to prevent or reverse weight gain and its complications, one needs to have a clear understanding of the root causes of the problem. At present, obesity research in the UK is highly esteemed and British workers feature prominently in World Congresses on obesity. Yet the economic imbalances described above suggest that a much greater investment in research into basic mechanisms is justifiable in Britain. In this paper I will therefore consider some of the evidence for the metabolic basis of obesity and assess the potential for new research.

THE PROBLEM OF THE WEIGHT:

Metabolic Factors, Energy Balance and Obesity

The principle of conservation of energy, applied to human energy balance, provides the commonplace assertion that the overweight must have consumed more energy - calories - than they should in order to remain thin. It also allows the usually painful corollary that in order to lose weight they must consume less than they expend. It is an absorbing question whether there is primary hyperphagia to create the initial energy surplus for weight gain or whether a small defect in energy expenditure is the main event. The data of Payne and Griffiths (1976) suggests that the non-obese, but perhaps pre-obese, children of obese parents tend to be less physically active and to take proportionately less food energy than children of non-obese parents, which may indicate that overeating is the primary decompensating event. Obese adults appear not to expend less energy than lean on physical exertion (Blair and Buskirk, 1987).

In either event, a failure of the other side of the energy balance equation is necessary to bypass the compensatory mechanisms that normally keep body weight constant. In its earliest stages at least obesity tends to develop gradually and this can be shown to result from tiny, almost imperceptible imbalances in the energy balance equation

$$\text{Energy intake} = \text{Energy expenditure} \pm \text{Change in energy stores.}$$

A persistent 1% error in energy balance would lead to weight gain of 1 - 2kg per year or about one stone in 5 years. Such tendencies would normally be compensated by changes in the opposite side of the equation. Herein lies the fundamental problem for research: whether an apparent defect has a primary aetiological role or whether it is a secondary development. It is not sufficient to simply demonstrate differences between obese and lean in order to speculate about why some people get fat, although there may be clues as to how they remain fat. The seductive search for a simple endocrine basis for obesity has been particularly fruitless in this respect, although there are several endocrine diseases where obesity develops and altered hormonal responses (adrenal, pancreatic, gonadal, thyroid or pituitary) may be found in obesity.

Energy Intake In Obesity

A large literature has built up, examining both energy intake and energy expenditure in relation to obesity. Much confusion has arisen because of the inherent difficulties in assessing the eating habits of the overweight. Most large surveys have failed to demonstrate overeating by the obese. Completely erroneous concepts abound such as that of "low energy throughput" from a survey by Keen et al (1979) of 3400 subjects using dietary record analysis which apparently demonstrated reduced energy intake in the overweight. It is not clear whether the obese systematically under-record food intake during such surveys, or whether they inevitably and subconsciously undereat for the period of the study. Either way, food intake is consistently underestimated by the overweight. Energy expenditure measured in absolute terms by calorimetry, and more recently in freeliving individuals using the doubly labelled water technique, is consistently elevated in the obese who must therefore be eating more to remain in energy balance (James et al, 1978; Jequier, 1984; Prentice et al, 1986).

Figure 2: DIET COMPOSITION AND BODY WEIGHT
Recalculated from West (1974) and West & Kalbfleisch (1971)

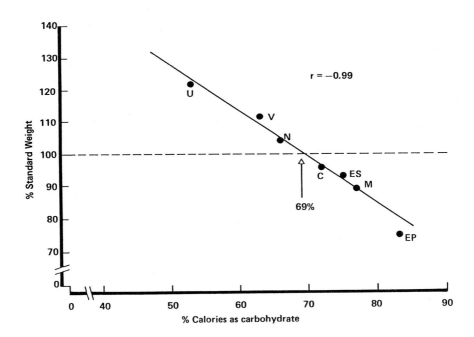

Given these difficulties in assessing energy intake in obesity, conclusions about the role of habitual dietary composition on the development of obesity must remain suspect. There is some epidemiological data between countries to suggest that obesity is less likely to develop with very high carbohydrate (thus low fat) intakes (Figure 2). Laboratory studies have shown that animals normally fed a high carbohydrate chow diet can become obese if given a cafeteria diet with a higher fat intake, and indeed there are differences between strains in the ease with which this happens. The addition of sucrose or ethanol also stimulates appetite and weight gain. Perhaps the most intriguing data are those of Lin and Romsos (1979) who demonstrated that congenitally obese mice have increased energetic efficiency and

4

gain weight faster on a high fat diet (80% energy) than on an isoenergetic low fat diet (20% energy). Control mice in the same experiment showed no such sensitivity to diet composition. Wade (1982) showed that hamsters could also gain weight without overeating when on a high fat diet, mainly by reducing energy expenditure while resting.

Energy Expenditure

In humans there are few studies of obesity-prone subjects, i.e. where the secondary effects of obesity can be excluded. Shetty et al, gave a 32% fat/45% carbohydrate/23% protein test meal to post-obese women and found a significantly reduced thermogenic response compared with controls (Shetty et al, 1981). Jequier and co-workers have also found reduced thermic responses over 3 hours following a mixed meal and also after a 100g glucose load in post-obese subjects compared to lean controls (Jequier & Schutz, 1985). Our data on the energetic effects of carbohydrate and fat feeding over 24 hours, described later, suggest that the post-obese can still respond to carbohydrate but that there is a significant defect, compared to controls, in thermic response to a mixed diet containing 40% fat/45% carbohydrate (Lean and James, 1987).

From animal evidence it might be suspected that altered catecholamine responses may lead to impaired thermogenic responses in the obesity-prone, perhaps interacting with altered thyroid or other hormonal responses to feeding. In experimental animals brown adipose tissue is the organ responsible for regulatory thermogenesis, but there is no suggestion that human brown adipose tissue plays a major role in diet-induced thermogenesis in adulthood although the tissue is still present and retains the potential for thermogenesis (Lean and James, 1986). There is some suggestion of reduced noradrenaline responsiveness in post-obese women (Jung et al, 1979) and also of impaired catecholamine, growth hormone and prolactin but exaggerated cortisol responses to insulin hypoglycaemia (Jung et al, 1982). Shetty et al, however, could demonstrate no simple endocrine abnormality in post-obese women to explain the reduced thermogenesis.

Energy intake remains perhaps the most critical arm of the energy balance equation for management in that it can be modified to a greater degree. The abnormality of appetite in obesity is that it is appropriate, given the foods available, to weight maintenance at an elevated level. Dietary intake can undoubtedly be reduced by modifying appetite in a number of ways but it is uncertain whether increased appetite is a primary cause of simple obesity apart from some rare pathological conditions such as the Prader Willi syndrome, or whether it is a secondary response to the increased body mass. However, it is necessary for the maintenance of obesity that appetite does not fall when weight gain occurs. Most adults actually maintain their body weight ± 10% effortlessly for 50 years, i.e. with 0.0001% accuracy. The way this fine balance is achieved remains elusive.

Animal studies point to a highly complicated regulation system centred on the hypothalamus and involving catecholaminergic, serotoninergic and peptidergic pathways. There is evidence for similar functions in man, but not of the primary defects which lead to obesity.

Basal Metabolism and Obesity

It is often suggested that people get fat because of "slow metabolism". As the largest component (c75%) of total energy expenditure, it is natural to look to the basal or resting metabolic rate for small differences between individuals which could have a large cumulative effect on energy balance. The resting energy expenditure is increased, not decreased in obesity. This has been clearly demonstrated. BMR is principally determined by the fat-free body mass which is also increased in obesity. Basal metabolism therefore falls with weight loss and most studies on post-obese subjects show very similar figures to those of lean controls. There is some suggestion that BMR in the post-obese may be lower when expressed per kg fat-free mass compared with well matched controls, so this may depend on the extend of weight loss (Lean and James, 1987). Bogardus et at (1986) found evidence for a genetic factor in basal metabolism, but it did not relate to a tendency to obesity.

The Genetics of Obesity

It is a common observation that being overweight runs in families but it is unclear whether this reflects a genetic basis or is the end result of a common family environment. Certain rare chromosomal defects are known to produce obesity as part of congenital syndromes. These may offer clues to mechanisms but do not relate to the inheritance of obesity in general. Overweight in children has a correlation of about 0.25 with one obese parent, perhaps suggesting a polygenic inheritance, and is progressively more frequent if both parents, and if grandparents are obese (Garn, 1986). However, the correlations between related adults are much less strong (Garn et al, 1981), and it is also known that synchronous changes in fatness occur in family members both of which point towards envirnonmental factors. Studies of twins show high concordance rates for degree of overweight with closer correlations between monozygotic than dizygotic twins. The heritable component is put at about 0.8, a higher heritability than for, say, hypertension or schizophrenia (0.6) or ischaemic heart disease (0.5) (Stunkard et al, 1986).

Comparison of the similarities between non-related individuals living together and related individuals exposed to different environments gives greater insight. Stunkard et at (1986) studied 540 Danish adoptees, as adults, and both their adoptive and biological parents. Significant relationships between the BMI of adoptees and biological parents, especially for mothers and daughters, were reported, but no relation was found with BMI of adoptive parents. The study relied on self-reporting and memory recall of heights and weights, but was blind in the sense that most adoptees had no knowledge of their biological parents and vice versa.

Bouchard and his colleagues in Quebec (1985) have recently

analysed large studies of siblings and families to examine the roles of genetic and environmental factors in determining obesity and fat distribution. Increasing similarity in fatness was observed between siblings, dizygotic and monozygotic twins, but none was detected between adoptive siblings. The greater heritability between dizygotic twins than between siblings must be reflecting environmental factors, since their gene similarity (50%) is identical. Genetic effects were found for the measurement of subcutaneous fat, fat distribution, body density and fat-free mass. The significance of environmental factors was highlighted by the similarities found between children and parents and between adoptive children and foster parents. Interclass correlations for BMI and skinfold thicknesses were almost identical, but extremity/trunk ratio and the proportion of total fat mass in subcutaneous sites were more closely correlated in natural than adoptive relations.

Interaction between Genetic and Environmental Influences

In addition to the evidence for genetic (G) and environmental (E) influences on the phenotypic (P) expression of fatness and fat distribution, Bouchard and colleagues propose another, interactive, factor (GxE)

$$VP = VG + VE + VGxE + e$$

where V denotes the variance and e the error variance (usually ignored).

Monozygotic twin studies by Poehlman et at (1986) using an overfeeding regime have shown significant GxE interactions for increase in body fat, fat mass and fat distribution. Biochemical markers such as lipoprotein lipase activity likewise showed GxE effects in response to overfeeding.

While it is exciting to be able to demonstrate that there is indeed an interactive factor and quantitate it mathematically, this work does not identify the specific dietary element responsible in overfeeding, from which one might make some nutritional deduction for the management or prevention of obesity. We have used a different approach towards identifying a specific "GxE" interaction. If one is now allowed to assume that obese subjects have a genetic predisposition towards increased energetic efficiency, and that this genetic factor remains after weight loss, it is possible to study the "GxE" effects of environmental factors i.e. different diets by comparing responses in post-obese compared with normal weight control subjects who are not prone to weight gain.

A total of 23 women were studied, 9 obese, 7 post-obese and 7 control, by whole body indirect calorimetry whilst in very precise energy balance. They were studied whilst consuming two isocaloric diets over 24 hours, a "low-fat" diet containing 3% of total energy as fat, 82% carbohydrate, and a "high-fat" diet with 40% fat, 45% carbohydrate designed to correspond closely to the average habitual diet. Thermogenic effects of the two diets were expressed through the increment of energy expenditure above that measured on a previous 24 hour fasting study using an identical supervised protocol, as a percentage of the fed energy expenditure. The results (Figure 3) showed a lower overall thermic effect from high-fat feeding than from the low fat/high carbohydrate diet, but the difference was only significant in the post-obese and ANOVA confirmed a significant interaction between subject group and diet.

Figure 3: RESPONSES OF CONTROLS, POST-OBESE AND OBESE WOMEN TO TWO ISOCALORIC DIETS

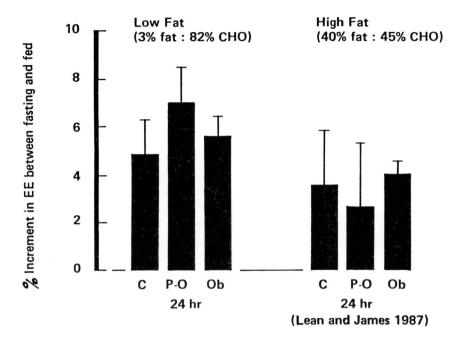

(Lean and James 1987)

These subjects were then studied on further occasions with the same high-fat diet supplemented with carbohydrate to 150% of energy balance. Multiple stepwise regression analyses of the three feeding regimes (low fat, high fat and overfed) indicated linear relationships between energy expenditure and carbohydrate intake which were significantly different in the control and post-obese groups ($p < 0.02$). Energy expenditure was lower in the post-obese group for the same carbohydrate intake when carbohydrate formed less then 70% of total energy requirement (Figure 4). No independent effect was detected of dietary fat on 24 hour energy expenditure in either group, but there was a significant negative correlation ($p < 0.05$) between fat intake and sleeping metabolic rate in the post-obese group which was not apparent in the controls.

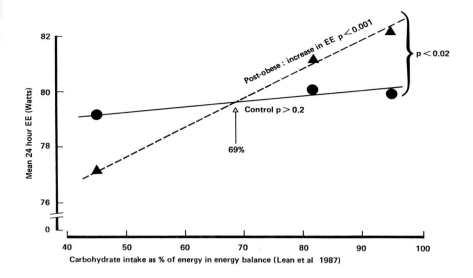

The size of the defect demonstrated in the post-obese group, on a 40% fat diet similar to that in the general population, was 1 - 2% of total energy intake. This approaches the limits of detection using even the highly sophisticated equipment now available to measure energy expenditure, but it would be enough to account for weight gain at a rate of around 2 - 3kg per annum and could be important in causing gradual weight gain provided it is not overcome by compensatory reduction in appetite.

Conclusion

Currently obesity research is being pursued with enthusiasm and producing results. It can be asserted with some confidence that obesity falls within the medical/biological concept of a disease, and is not simply self-induced. Overeating above those requirements needed for maintaining a thin weight is obviously necessary for obesity to develop but attention is now being focussed on the reasons for this inadvertent imbalance. A person who gets fat has either a family history of overweight or alternatively a genetic combination which dictates an inherited bias towards obesity. The expression of this genetic background is facilitated by eating an habitual diet which contains too little carbohydrate and too much fat. Other "GxE" interactions may hitherto come to light but, at present, the high carbohydrate, high fibre, low fat diet together with regular, moderate exercise, seems increasingly justifiable as the most appropriate starting point for lifelong obesity management. Slimming diets based on these principles hold the best theoretical promise for long term success and are already used empirically by the largest and most successful slimming clubs. The final judgement on this dietary approach will depend on whether the combination of advantages to be expected of this type of diet i.e. reduced risk factors for disease, especially ischaemic heart disease, and now, possibly, better weight maintenance will result in better long term health than the multitude of "quick slim", short term approaches currently being advertised and so widely used.

Figure 5: THE ENERGY CYCLE

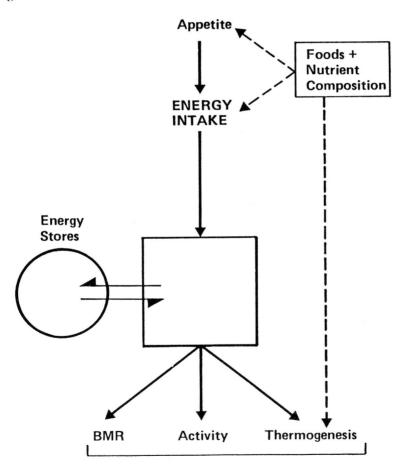

References

1. Blair D and Buskirk ER. Habitual daily energy expenditure and activity levels of lean and adult-onset and child-onset obese women. Am J Clin Nutr 1987; *45:* 540-545.

2. Bogardus C, Lilloja S, Ravussin E, Abbott W, Zawadziki JK, Young A, Knowler WC, Jacobowitz R and Moll PP. Familial dependence of the resting metabolic rate. New Eng J Med 1986; *315:* 96-100.

3. Bouchard C. Inheritance of fat distribution and adipose tissue metabolism. In, Metabolic Complications of the Human Obesities, eds. Vague J, Bjorntorp P, Guy-Grand B, Rebuffe-Scrive M and Vague Ph Elsevier: Amsterdam 1985: 87-96.

4. Bouchard C, Savard R, Despres J-P, Tremblay A and Leblanc C. Body composition in adopted and biological siblings. Hum Biol 1985; *57:* 61-75.

5. Flatt JP. Energetics of intermediary metabolism. In, Eds. Garrow JS and Halliday D. Substrate and Energy Metabolism. John Libbey: London, 1985: 58-69.

6. Garn SM. The genetics of obesity. Nutr Reviews 1986; *44:* 381-386.

7. Garn SM, Bailey SM, Solomon BA, and Hopkins PJ. Effect of remaining family members on fatness prediction. AM J Clin Nutr 1981; *34:* 148-153.

8. James WPT, Bailes J, Davies HL, and Dauncey MJ. Elevated metabolic rates in obesity. Lancet 1978; *i:* 1122-1125.

9. Jequier E. Energy expenditure in obesity. Clin Endocrinol Metab 1984; *13:* 563-580.

10. Jequier E, and Schutz Y. Recent Advances in Obesity Research, IV, ed Hirsch J and van Itallie TB. John Libbey: London, 1985: 76-81.

11. Jung RT, Shetty PS, James WPT, Barrand MA and Callingham BA. Reduced thermogenesis in obesity. Nature 1979; *279:* 322-323.

12. Jung RT, Campbell RG, James WPT and Callingham BA. Altered hypothalamic and sympathetic responses to hypoglycaemia in familial obesity. Lancet 1982; *i:* 1043-1046.

13. Keen H, Thomas BJ, Jarret RJ and Fuller JH. Nutrient intake, adiposity and diabetes. Br Med J 1979; *i:* 655-658.

14. Laing WA. The cost of diet related diseases. In, Preventive Nutrition and Society, ed. Turner MR, Academic Press: London 1981: 55-76.

15. Lean MEJ and James WPT. Brown adipose tissue in man. In, Brown Adipose Tissue, eds, Trayhurn P and Nicholls DG, Edward Arnold: London, 1986: 339-366.

16. Lean MEJ and James WPT. Metabolic effects of isoenergetic nutrient exchange over 24 hours in relation to obesity in women. Int J Obesity 1987; in press.

17. Lin P-Y, Romsos DR, Vander Tuig JG and Leveille GA. Maintenance energy requirements, energy retention and heat production of young obese (ob ob) and lean mice fed a high-fat or a high-carbohydrate diet. J Nutr 1979; *109:* 1143-1153.

18. Payne PR and Griffiths M. Energy expenditure in small children of obese and non-obese parents. Nature 1976; *260:* 698-700.

19. Poehlman ET, Tremblay A, Despres J-P, Fontaine E, Perusse L, Theriault G and Bouchard C. Genotype-controlled changes in body composition and fat morphology following overfeeding in twins. Am J Clin Nutr 1986 *43:* 723-731.

20. Poehlman ET, Despres J-P, Marcotte M, Tremblay A, Theriault G and Bouchard C. Genotype dependency of adaptation in adipose tissue metabolism after short-term overfeeding. Am J Physiol 1986; *250:* (Endocrinol Metab 13) E480-485.

21. Prentice AM, Black AE, Coward WA, Davies HL, Goldberg GR, Murgatroyd PR, Ashford H, Sawyer M and Whitehead RG. High levels of energy expenditure in obesity. Br Med J 1986 *292:* 983-987.

22. Shetty PS, Jung RT, James WPT, Barrand MA and Callingham BA. Post-prandial thermogenesis in obesity. Clin Sci 1981; *60:* 519-525.

23. Stunkard AJ, Foch TT and Hrubec Z. A twin study of human obesity. J A M A 1986; *256:* 51-54.

24. Stunkard AJ, Sorensen TIA, Hanis C, Teasdale YW, Chakraborty R, Schull WJ and Schulsinger F. An adoption study of human obesity. New Engl J Med 1986; *314:* 193-198.

25. Wade GN. Obesity without overeating in golden hamsters. Physiol Behav 1982; *29:* 701-707.

26. West KM. Epidemiology of Diabetes and its Vascular Lesions. Elsevier: New York, 1978.

27. West KM and Kalbfleisch JM. Influence of nutritional factors on prevalence of diabetes. Diabetes 1971; *20:* 99-108.

GIP-THE OBESITY HORMONE

V Marks

Professor of Clinical Biochemistry
University of Surrey, Guildford

Introduction

"It's my glands doctor" has long been the cry of the morbidly obese who, despite doing everything they can, stubbornly refuse to lose weight. It is indeed true that some endocrine diseases are associated with morbid obesity but, in very few of them, is it the sole or even most important feature and few students of obesity put much store by claims that a patient's obesity owes more to his/her endocrine make-up than to gluttony or at least inadvertant overeating (Dieguez and Scanlon 1987).

Endocrine Causes of Obesity

The insulinoma syndrome has long been known to be associated with gross obesity but when it does occur it is usually iatrogenic, developing only as a consequence of patients being advised to eat in order to delay, or prevent, the appearance of neuroglycopenic symptoms. Nevertheless patients do, from time to time, present with obesity, seemingly of the simple variety, in whom an insulinoma can be shown to be the sole causative agent, and yet who do not experience neuroglycopenia except in response to prolonged fasting or the institution of very low energy dietary intake (Labib et at 1987). In such patients removal of the tumour can, as in one patient of my own, lead to loss of 25Kg in weight in just four months without recourse to excessively strict or socially unacceptable dieting. Obesity occurring either antenatally or during the first few weeks of life is common in another form of primary hyperinsulinism namely that due to nesidioblastosis or functional hyperinsulinism of infancy (Marks & Rose 1981). Like the hypoglycaemia - which is the hallmark of the disease - the obesity of nesidioblastosis responds dramatically to treatment aimed at reducing the hyperinsulinism.

Both insulinoma and nesidioblastosis are exceedingly rare conditions and represent only an infinitesimal proportion of all patients suffering from obesity. Moreover they are characterised by inappropriate insulin secretion i.e. failure of insulin secretion to suppress in response to hypoglycaemia, rather than to excessive insulin secretion, more typically seen in patients with "insulin resistance" and/or "simple obesity". They are, however, but one end of a spectrum which links obesity and states of altered insulin secretion.

Insulin and Obesity

It has long been known that exogenous insulin administered

experimentally to animals and therapeutically to man can, if excessive, cause obesity (Marks & Davidson 1976).

Soon after the invention of radioimmunoassay it was established that the single most characteristic clinical biochemical feature of obesity, regardless of its primary aetiology, is hyperinsulinaemia. Obese subjects not only have high overnight fasting plasma insulin levels compared with normal weight subjects but also show exaggerated insulinaemic responses to the majority of insulin-secretory stimuli (Marks & Samols 1968). The hyperinsulinaemia of "simple" obesity differs, however, from that of insulinoma and nesidioblastosis in that it is never inappropriate i.e. it does not induce spontaneous hypoglycaemia or endure in its presence.

The question of whether hyperinsulinaemia is the cause, or the effect, of obesity has troubled investigators since the association between obesity and hyperinsulinism was first discovered. Abstention from food or gross reduction in caloric intake by obese subjects for more than a relatively short period reduces or abolishes the exaggerated islet B-cell response to insulinotrophic stimuli and lowers the normally high basal insulin levels usually observed in these subjects even though bodyweight loss has been minimal (Marks and Samols 1968). This suggests that food intake rather than body mass is the main determining factor in the hyperinsulinaemia of obesity though other factors are undoubtedly involved.

Entero-Insular Axis

Prior to 1964 it was generally assumed that the major, if not sole, stimulus to insulin secretion by the pancreas was the arterial blood glucose concentration. In a brilliant piece of investigative work MacIntyre, Holdsworth & Turner (1964) showed that, when given by the enteral route, glucose was much more insulin stimulatory than when given intravenously so as to produce similar or greater degrees of arterial hyperglycaemia. The authors postulated that nutrients taken by mouth stimulate the release of one or more hormones which, in turn, augment glucose-stimulated insulin release. Such a substance had previously been postulated and tentatively called "incretin" by Zuntz and La Barre but the search for it had been abandoned after their existence had been reputedly, but wrongly, disproved. The renewed search for, and identification of, "incretin" began with the independent discoveries in London by ourselves that glucagon is an extremely potent stimulus to insulin secretion (Samols et at 1965) and by Dupre (1964) that commercially available preparations of (impure) secretin could, under certain circumstances, stimulate insulin secretion but above all, by the demonstration by McIntyre et at (1964) of the alimentary augmentation of insulin secretion.

GIP (Gastric Inhibitory Peptide)

Further work by numerous investigators throughout the world (summarised by Marks & Turner 1977) led eventually to the conclusion

14

that, amongst the known gastrointestinal hormones, GIP has the strongest claim to be considered the hypothetical "incretin". GIP was the name given to a substance, first isolated by Dr. John Brown working in the laboratories of Professor Victor Mutt in Stockholm, whose activity was characterised by its potent inhibitory effect upon gastric acid secretion (Brown 1982). Not until some three or so years later was its insulin stimulatory properties identified.

GIP - also known as gastric inhibitory polypeptide, glucose dependent insulin-stimulatory peptide, or preferably, GIP - is a 42 amino-acid, single-chain polypeptide secreted by endocrine cells sited in the intestinal mucosa. There are small interspecies differences between GIPs from different species. The first GIP to be isolated and characterised was that obtained from the pig and most investigations into the pharmacology of GIP have been carried out using this compound. Porcine GIP differs from human GIP by a single amino-acid but this is sufficient, in some cases, to produce important differences in biological and immunological properties. This fact has only recently come to light and explains some of the seemingly incompatible or frankly contradictory results obtained by different workers using atypical materials or reagents.

GIP can be measured in biological fluids by radioimmunoassay, usually employing an antiserum raised against porcine GIP with complete cross-reactivity against human GIP (Morgan et al 1976). Immunoreactive GIP occurs in plasma in two forms; the most prevalent form has a molecular weight of 5,000 daltons and corresponds to GIP as isolated from the gut; the other form has an apparent molecular weight of 8,000 daltons and is of unknown origin, function and composition. Only the 5,000 dalton material is justifiable referred to as GIP.

Regulation of GIP Secretion

GIP secretion is stimulated by the ingestion of carbohydrates after their conversion into actively absorbed sugars such as glucose and galactose. It is not stimulated by passively absorbed sugars, such as fructose, or by polyols, such as xylitol, nor is it stimulated by glucose whose active transport has been blocked by phloridzin (Sykes et at 1977). Long chain fatty acids, but not short or medium chain fatty acids, are equal or more powerful stimuli to GIP secretion than equimolar amounts of carbohydrate, as are triglycerides which are normally hydrolysed to long chain fatty acids and monoglycerides in the bowel (Kwasowski et al 1985). Patients with exocrine pancreatic failure who are unable to hydrolise triglycerides do not show the normal GIPaemic response to the ingestion of triglycerides but do so if given with lipase by mouth (Brown 1982).

Like carbohydrate-induced GIP secretion, fat-stimulated GIP is, in some way, linked to its active absorption and to the production of chylomicrons. Short and medium chain fatty acids that are not packaged by mucosal cells into chylomicrons but are instead secreted straight into the portal venous circulation do not stimulate GIP secretion . Proteins and amino acids are poor stimuli to GIP secretion and alcohol is completely without effect.

A negative feedback control by insulin upon fat-stimulated GIP secretion can ordinarily be demonstrated in human beings. There is some evidence, from rat studies, that the C-peptide of proinsulin exerts a similar inhibitory effect upon fat-stimulated GIP secretion (Dryburgh et al 1980). The inhibitory effect of insulin upon fat-stimulated GIP secretion can be attenuated by prior high fat feeding, both in human beings and laboratory animals, and attenuation occurs naturally in people consuming a high fat diet. A similar attenuation of insulin feedback control of fat stimulated GIP secretion is seen in most obese subjects - whether diabetic or not: indeed diabetes itself seems to be largely irrelevant to the control of GIP secretion except indirectly through insulin availability. Insulin does not exert negative feedback control on carbohydrate induced GIP secretion serving yet again to distinguish between the two major classes of stimuli to GIP secretion.

Pharmacological properties of GIP

Although named for its ability to inhibit gastric acid secretion GIP has attracted most interest in biology because of its potent insulin stimulatory properties. These insulinotropic effects are, however, manifested only in the presence of mild to moderate hyperglycaemia (Brown 1982). Consequently the GIP released from the gut in response to triglyceride ingestion, for example, does not, in normal healthy subjects produce a rise in plasma insulin concentration. When, however, a complex meal providing both carbohydrate and fat is eaten the effect upon insulin secretion is much greater than can be accounted for solely by the rise in arterial blood glucose concentration. This situation can be mimicked experimentally, for example, by the ingestion, during the course of an intravenous glucose infusion, of either fat or galactose - both of which stimulate GIP and insulin secretion under these circumstances but which have no or very little insulin-stimulatory properties in their own right (Morgan et al 1979).

In addition to its effect upon insulin secretion in the fed state, GIP activates liprotein lipase and hastens chylomicron clearance from the circulation by adipocytes (Eckel et al 1979; Wasada et al 1981). It also modulates insulin action on both the liver (Hartman et al 1986) and adipose tissue (Starich et al 1985) increasing its biological effects and encouraging the uptake of glucose by hepatocytes and adipocytes. It is possible to speculate, therefore, that a hormone possessing the properties of GIP (namely one with the ability to stimulate insulin, but only after the ingestion of food, and to favour direct uptake of dietary fat into the main energy storage tissue i.e. the adipocytes of white fat) would have important survival value for animals, such as man, whose access to food might be seasonal. Such a hormone would favour the deposition and storage of fat in times of plenty but have no adverse effects during famine. This hypothesis, which is supported by a large body of evidence - only some of which it is possible to present at this time - is compatible with evidence linking the ability to become obese, when food is plentiful, with genetic inheritance (Stunkard et al 1986).

GIP and Obesity

The first intimation that GIP production and secretion might be deranged in obesity came from observations made in my laboratory that mice with hereditary obesity (ob/ob) had much larger amounts of GIP in their gut mucosa than did their thin litter mates (Polak et al 1975; Bailey et al 1986). These mice - homozygous for the ob gene - have long been recognised as being grossly hyperinsulinaemic as well as mildy hyperglycaemic. It was subsequently shown, mainly by Creutzfeld and co-workers in Germany, that obese human subjects, whether diabetic or not, have exaggerated plasma GIP responses to enteric glucose or fat. Another fact to emerge, of possibly even great aetiologic significance, is that obese individuals generally fail to show the normal inhibitory effect of insulin upon fat stimulated GIP secretion (Brown 1982). A similar insensitivity to negative feed-back control by insulin upon GIP secretion can be induced in healthy, normal-weight subjects by feeding them a high fat diet for a month or so (Morgan 1983; Morgan et al 1987).

Fat-Feeding, Experimental Obesity and GIP Secretion

Experimentally, animals fed various "confectionery style" diets, differing in composition but not in total energy, showed induction of GIP production and secretion in response to diets that are high in fat but not to diets that are high in sugar content (Bailey et al 1986). Weight gain is significantly greater in animals fed a high fat diet than those fed an equi-caloric high sugar diet. The difference between the GIP inducing properties of fat and sugar cafeteria diets, originally observed in genetically obese mice, can also be demonstrated in normal weight rats (Tan et al 1987).

Experiments on healthy normal weight human volunteers have shown (Morgan et al 1987) that after consumption of a fat supplemented diet for one month plasma GIP responses to standard oral carbohydrate and fat loads are exaggerated and the normal inhibitory effect of exogenous insulin upon fat-stimulated GIP release is attenuated (Morgan et al 1987). Thus amongst energy providing foods long chain triglycerides currently seem uniquely able to induce non-insulin suppressable hypergipaemia. This in turn may play a role in the hyperinsulinaemia observed in such conditions as obesity where normal feedback control by insulin upon fat-induced GIP secretion is known to be deranged.

Hypothesis

The postulated role for GIP in the production of obesity is summarised in Figure 1. Briefly it is considered to provide a mechanism whereby excess energy intake over and above daily requirements can be most efficiently stored against times of food deprivation rather than being wastefully oxidised through thermogenesis.

Figure 1: THE ROLE OF GIP IN THE PRODUCTION OF OBESITY

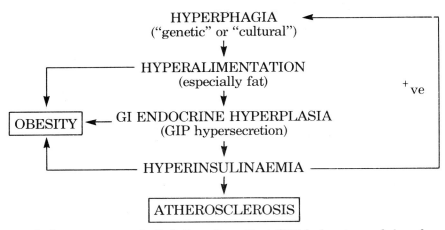

It is our current belief, therefore, that GIP helps to explain why energy derived from long-chain triglycerides appears to be "more fattening" than that derived from other sources - notably carbohydrates, proteins and alcohol - all of which must undergo energy requiring transformations before being deposited as fat. Moreover since insulin itself is atherogenic (Stout 1987) the intervention of GIP and its induction by high fat feeding, may help to explain why high fat diets are more atherogenic than high carbohydrate diets - especially those rich in soluble fibre content - without invoking the "cholesterol" hypothesis which is far from completely convincing.

Summary

GIP is an "anabolic" hormone which functions only under certain dietary conditions, namely during the absorption of food. It stimulates the release of insulin in the presence of mild to moderate hyperglycaemia such as that which follows the ingestion of a mixed meal and it favours the uptake of exogenous fat by adipose tissue. GIP production is increased in obese subjects and experimental animals. Its production and secretion is inducible by high fat feeding. It is postulated that a hormone possessing GIP properties would be expected to favour the development of obesity in hyperalimented subjects and that GIP might provide the link between genetic programming for obesity and its manifestation in life.

References

1. Bailey CJ, Flatt PR, Kwasowski P, Powell CJ and Marks V. Immunoreactive gastric inhibitory polypeptide and K cell hyperplasia in obese hyperglycaemic (ob/ob) mice fed high fat and high carbohydrate cafeteria diets. Acta Endocrinologica 1986; *112*: 224-229.
2. Brown JC. Gastric inhibitory polypeptide. Berlin: Spinger-Verlag, 1982:88.
3. Diegulez C, Scanlon MF. The search for a hormonal switch for obesity. Br Med J 1987; *294*: 1371-1372.

4. Dupre J. An intestinal hormone affecting glucose disposal in man. Lancet 1964; ii, 672.

5. Dryburgh JR, Hampton SM and Marks V. Endocrine pancreatic control of the release of gastric inhibitory polypeptide: a possible physiological role for C-peptide. Diabetologia 1980; *19:* 397-401.

6. Eckel RH, Fujimoto WJ, Brunzell JD. Gastric inhibitory polypeptide enhances lipoprotein lipase activity in cultured pre-adipocytes. Diabetes 1979; *28:* 1141-1142.

7. Hartman H, Ebert R, Creutzfeldt W. Insulin dependent inhibition of hepatic glycogenolysis by gastric inhibitory polypeptide (GIP) in perfused rat liver. Diabetologia 1986; *29:* 112-114.

8. Kwasowski P, Flatt PR, Bailey CJ and Marks V. Effects of fatty acid chain length and saturation on gastric inhibitory polypeptide release in obese hyperglycaemic (ob/ob) mice. Bioscience Reports 1985; *5:* 701-705.

9. Labib M, Marks V, Patten J, Barker P, Laurent S and Boulter P. Insulinoma unmasked by the Cambridge Diet. Br Med J 1987; *294:* 1383-1384.

10. McIntyre N, Holdsworth D and Turner DS. New interpretation of oral glucose tolerance. Lancet 1964; *ii:* 20-21.

11. Marks HE and Davidson C. Hyperinsulinemia: effects on body weight, obesity and motivated behaviour. TIT, J Life Sci 1976, *6:* 1-10.

12. Marks V and Rose FC. Hypoglycaenia 2nd Edit. Oxford: Blackwell 1986.

13. Marks V and Samols E. Les taux plasmatiques d' hormones peptideques dans l'obesite: insuline, hormone de croissance et glucagon. Rev Med 1968; *21:* 1373-1382.

14. Samols E, Marri G and Marks V. Promotion of insulin secretion by glucagon. Lancet 1965: *2:* 415-416.

15. Marks V and Turner DS. The gastrointestinal hormones with particular reference to their role in the regulation of insulin secretion. Essays Med Biochem 1977: *3:* 109-152.

16. Morgan LM, Morris BA and Marks V. Radioimmunoassay of gastric inhibitory polypeptide Ann Clin Biochem 1978; *15:* 172-177.

17. Morgan LM. Wright JW and Marks V. The effect of oral galactose on GIP and insulin secretion in man. Diabetologia 1979; *16:* 235-239.

18. Morgan LM, Tredger JA, Hampton SM, Kwasowski P, Wright J, Dunne M and Marks V. Effect of diet upon response to oral fat and glucose in man; modification in control of the enteroinsular axis. Scand J Gastroenterol 1983; *18:* 99-101.

19. Morgan LM, Hampton SM, Tredger JA, Cramb R and Marks V. Modification of GIP secretion in man by a high fat diet; effect on the entero-insular axis (1987) submitted for publication.

20. Polak JM, Pearse AGE, Grimelius L and Marks V. Gastrointestinal apudosis in obese hyperglycaemic mice. Virchows Arch B Cell Path 1975; *19:* 135-150.

21. Starich GH, Bar RS and Mazzaferri EL. GIP increases insulin receptor affinity and cellular sensitivity in adipocytes. Am J Physiol 1985; *25G:* 603-607.

22. Stout RW. Insulin and atheroma - an update. Lancet 1987; *i:* 1077-1079.

23. Stunkard AJ, Sorensen TIA, Hanis C, Teasdale TW, Chakraborty R, Schull WJ and Schulsinger F. An adoption study of human obesity. New Engl J Med 1986; *314:* 193-197.

24. Sykes S, Morgan LM, English J and Marks V. Evidence for preferential stimulation of gastric inhibitory polypeptide secretion in the rat by actively transported carbohydrates. J Endocr 1980; *85:* 201-207.

25. Tan KS, Kwasowski P and Marks V. Effects of high fat cafeteria diet on plasma insulin (IRI) and gastric inhibitory polypeptide (IR-GIP) responses to a glucose load in the rat. Clin Sci 1987; *73:* 57p.

26. Wasada T, McCorkle C, Harris C, Kawai K, Howard B and Unger RH. Effect of gastric inhibitory polypeptide on plasma levels of chylomicron triglycerides in dogs. J Clin Invest 1981; *68:* 1106-1007.

Discussion

James: Increased food intake may be stimulating GIP which, in turn, enhances insulin output and sets in train the vicious cycle. In your volunteers did you keep their calorie intake the same?

Marks: No. They increased their food intake. The idea was to ensure that they were on a high fat intake. We achieved this be giving them an extra 70g fat per day in the form of double cream.

James: Therefore you had excess food intake in your human volunteers; presumably the fat mice were hyperphagic.

Marks: They were indeed hyperphagic and this is why we had to use the hyperphagic obese model as the control. We believe you have to have an increased food intake over energy expenditure in order to become obese but that not everyone experiences the same degree of GIP induction.

James: So your proposition is that whether you are a mouse or a man if you have an increase in food intake then there is a differential response in GIP depending on your genetic predisposition.

Marks: We believe that genes determine GIP production and secretion to a certain extent but so too does the nature of the diet. Fat is more GIPaemic than carbohydrate.

James: Have you shown that with isocaloric intakes of fat and carbohydrate?

Marks: In fact the diets fed to the obese animals were isocaloric but they put on more weight with the high fat diet than with the high carbohydrate diet.

Audience: What role does brown adipose tissue play in keeping a person thin. Do those who genetically have more brown adipose tissue remain thin?

Marks: Brown adipose tissue is an irrelevance in man. In rats it is very important in thermogenesis but it is of little significance in humans.

Audience: Are the K-cells which produce GIP universally distributed through the intestine?

Marks: They are mainly found in the duodenum, jejunum and to a very much lesser extent in the ileum. The maldistribution in the ob/ob mouse was striking in that there was a tremendous increase in ileal GIP cells.

Audience: Gastric bypass surgery should therefore be beneficial according to your theory?

Marks: Work has been published to show that GIP levels decrease in response to food if you bypass the most GIPaemic part of the gut.

THE SEARCH FOR THERMOGENIC DRUGS

M A Cawthorne

Beechams Pharmaceuticals Research Division,
Great Burgh, Epsom, Surrey

Introduction

Body weight is maintained constant when daily energy intake in the form of nutrients is matched by daily energy expenditure. To lose weight, one must either reduce energy intake or increase energy expenditure.

Pharmacotherapy for obesity has traditionally focussed on agents that affect appetite. Such agents have often failed to demonstrate long-term weight loss (Scoville, 1973). Two major approaches have been adopted in recent years to obtain greater and more prolonged weight loss. The first of these is to use low calorie diets and the second is to find ways of increasing energy expenditure. The most obvious way to increase energy expenditure is to take more exercise. There is much published work showing that exercise in rats will produce a marked anti-obesity effect, the weight loss being principally due to loss of fat. By contrast, weight loss resulting from dietary restriction produces a reduction in all body components (Wilson, Smith and Cawthorne, 1984). In man, the value of exercise as a treatment for obesity has proved difficult to substantiate but it is likely that the energy cost of exercise extends well beyond the period of activity into the post-exercise oxygen debt period. The available evidence suggests that the most successful form of exercise for weight reduction is aerobic daily exercise such as running for substantial periods at 70% of Vo2max. Unfortunately, in severely obese subjects such a form of exercise may be impossible. Another way to increase energy expenditure is by the use of drugs that stimulate metabolic rate. The objective of this paper is to review the search for safe thermogenic drugs.

Thyroid Hormones

Thyroid hormones were first used for the treatment of obesity in 1893 but their use is now limited to situations where replacement therapy is indicated. Much of the weight loss induced by thyroid hormone is protein rather than fat (Abraham et al, 1985) and a further disadvantage is that thyroid hormones affect cardiac function and increase the already high load imposed on the heart of obese subjects.

Uncoupling Agents

The first synthetic thermogenic drug to be introduced specifically for the treatment of obesity was dinitrophenol. It was introduced in 1933 and, over the following three years, more than 100,000 patients were treated. Whilst it was very effective, side-effects were common and serious including severe neurological defects, cataracts and some deaths.

Dinitrophenol increases metabolic rate by uncoupling the oxidative combustion of foods from ATP production. It seems probable that this mechanism of action, which is at the fulcrum of energy metabolism, is responsible for some of the serious side-effects and even the deaths caused by dinitrophenol. ATP, as the ultimate and essential energy source cannot have its production blocked without disasterous consequences.

Development of Screening Systems for Thermogenic Agents.

The search for thermogenic agents has been hindered by the lack of a suitable test system in animals. Miller and Stock (1969) suggested that one could detect thermogenic agents by doing energy balance experiments in rats. Thus, rats were fed on a diet containing a drug for 7 days and the total amount of food eaten was measured. Duing the experiment faeces and urine were collected and at the end of the experiment the animals were killed. The calorific values of the ingested food, the faeces, the urine and the carcasses were all measured using a ballistic bomb calorimeter. In addition, the calorific value of control animals, which had been killed at the beginning of the experiment, was also measured. From these data, Miller and Stock were able to calculate the amount of missing energy, and clearly any drug that increased this missing energy, which is equivalent to the metabolic rate of the animals, is potentially an anti-obesity agent. Although this method is considered to be the 'gold standard', it is time-consuming and labour intensive for a primary screen and a more rapid screening procedure is required.

Metablic rate can be derived from the measurement of oxygen consumption. The simplest system is one designed by Haldane at the turn of the century in which the oxygen consumed by an animal is estimated by weighing. The method is rather insensitive and it is only possible to obtain a single measure over a period of several hours. Thus, a highly potent but short-acting agent might be missed. Two different tupes of continuous recording systems have been developed. The first is a close-circuit system (Stock, 1966) in which animals are placed in an airtight box equipped with an absorbent for carbon dioxide and a pressure detector. The utilisation of oxygen by the animal results in a fall in the gas pressure in the chamber which is detected and, via a transducer, activates a gas-tight syringe to deliver pure oxygen until atmospheric pressure is restored. The whole system can be automated with on-line analysis of data. It is extremely sensitive and very suitable for monitoring rapid changes in energy expenditure over a period of a few hours. It is less suitable for more prolonged studies. The second system for testing the metabolic rate response to drugs evolved from collaboration between Derek Miller and the author (Boroumand and Miller, 1977; Arch et al, 1982). It is an adaption of the human open-circuit indirect calorimetry system and involves the measurement of the oxygen content of the expired air of animals using a paramagnetic oxygen analyser. Thus, by a knowledge of the flow rate of air through the animals cage, oxygen consumption can be measured continuously for periods up to several days and the metabolic rate derived from this. Adaptations of this latter system are used by a number of pharmaceutical companies for detecting thermogenic agents.

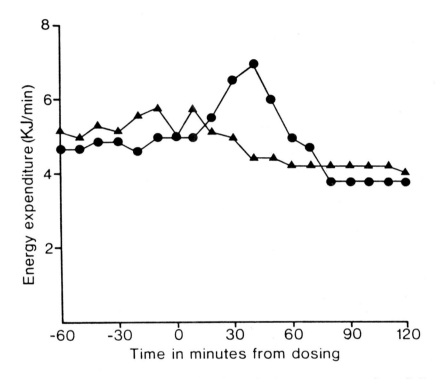

Figure 1: The effect of caffeinated and decaffeinated coffee on energy expenditure. Coffee was given at time 0 min. ●, caffeinated coffee; ▲, decaffeinated coffee.

Thermogenic Agents in Everyday Life

Caffeine (and other methylxanthines in coffee, tea, chocolate and coca-cola), alcohol and tobacco have all been shown to be thermogenic in some circumstances (Miller, 1974), but the compound that has attracted most attention is caffeine. There is no doubt that it is thermogenic in both laboratory animals and man - indeed a cup of coffee produces a significant increase in metabolic rate relative to an equivalent cup of decaffeinated coffee (Holland et al, 1981) see Figure 1. However, the thermic effect of caffeine is short-lived and its effects, and those of its closely related xanthine, theophylline, in reducing fat deposition in rats and mice are usually small. There are no reports of caffeine having anti-obesity effects in man. Arch et al (1987) have suggested that the failure of caffeine to induce an anti-obesity effect may be because its short-term stimulant effect on metabolic rate is followed by a compensatory depression of metabolic rate.

Sympathomimetic Agents

Phenylpropanolamines and N-methyl phenylpropanolamines such as ephedrine are sympathomimetic agents that have long-established anorectic properties. The anorectic effect of ephedrine has been assumed to account for the loss of body weight produced in man by 'Elsinore pills' (Malchow-Moller et al, 1981). However, energy balance studies in mice have shown that ephedrine reduces body weight and fat content by a mechanism other than, or additional to, reduced food intake. Its thermogenic activity has subsequently been demonstrated in rodents and in man. The effect of ephedrine is believed to be a consequence of noradrenaline release leading to thermogenesis in brown adipose tissue (Wellman and Marmon, 1985) and skeletal muscle (Astrup et al, 1985). The release of noradrenaline induced by sympathomimetics occurs widely throughout the body and the endogenous noradrenaline can act at a wide-variety of adrenergic receptors. Thus, it would be surprising if thermogenesis leading to weight loss could be achieved in man without side-effects. In fact, clinical studies on ephedrine have produced equivocal and disappointing results (Pasquali et al, 1985, 1987).

Xanthine - Sympathomimetic Agent Combination

Miller (1974) was the first to note that caffeine potentiated the thermic effect of food and subsequent studies have shown that it potentiates also the thermogenic action of ephedrine in rodents and man (Dulloo and Miller, 1986 a and b; Wellman and Marmon, 1985). The former authors also found significant differences between naturally lean subjects and lean subjects who had been previously obese and only maintained their body weight by dieting. In the post-obest subjects, the ephedrine/methylxanthine combination produced both a reduction in food intake and an increase in energy expenditure. Both these effects were absent in the lean subjects.

Clinical evaluation of ephedrine-methylxanthine combinations as anti-obesity treatments has not been widely undertaken but in the one study undertaken it was as effective as the anorectic drug ephedine (Malchow-Moller et at, 1981).

Beta-adrenoceptor Agonists

Sympathomimetic agents such as ephedrine produce a non-selective activation of the sympathetic nervous system resulting in a stimulation of all types of adrenoceptor. This mechanism is not attractive to those seeking a thermogenic anti-obesity agent since it is likely to cause side-effects that are not essentially linked to thermogenesis. In particular, alpha-adrenoceptor stimulation increases blood pressure and stimulates the central nervous system. Thermogenesis on the other hand is primarily mediated by beta-adrenoceptor stimulation and this receptor can be differentiated in rodents from those receptors associated with atrial stimulation (β_1) and uterine contraction (β_2) (Arch et al, 1984). This finding has led a number of research groups to develop novel selective beta-adrenoceptor agonists as potential thermogenic anti-obesity agents (Arch et al, 1984; Meier et al, 1984; Yen et al, 1984).

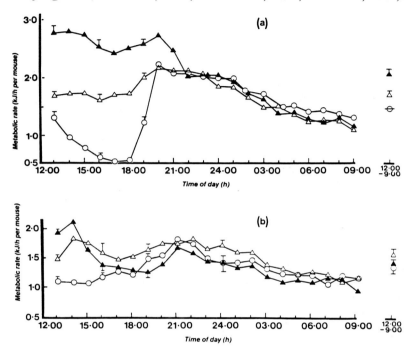

Figure 2: *Effect of repeat dosing BRL 26830A (0.2 mg per mouse per day) on metabolic rate of (a) obese and (b) lean C57BL/6 mice at 23.5°C.* The metabolic rate of the obese mice was measured[2] after the 18th dose of water (○), after the 18th dose of BRL 26830A (▲) or after the 1st dose of BRL 26830A when water had been given on the preceding 17 days (△). Mean body weights were: water, 40 g; BRL 26830A, day 18, 37 g; BRL 26830A, day 1, 39 g. The metabolic rate of the lean mice was measured after the 8th dose of water (○), after the 8th dose of BRL 26830A (▲) or after the 1st dose of BRL 26830A when water had been given on the preceding 7 days (△). Mean body weights were 24 g for each group of lean mice. The treatments were given at 1200 h. The dark period was 1800-0600 h. *n*=4.

Arch et al (1984) showed that one of these agents, BRL 26830A, selectively stimulates thermogenesis in vivo (Figure 2) and this action increases upon repeat dosing in obese rodents. In anti-obesity studies in obese rodents, BRL 26830A produced a selective loss of lipid with no reduction in lean body mass (Figure 3). The compound had no effect on the body weight in lean animals. Temporal studies show that initially there is a marked thermogenic response in lean animals but this is rapidly attenuated. Thus, it appears that BRL 26803A allows a natural mechanism to operate to prevent depletion of lipid stores in lean animals. In addition to its anti-obesity action, this compound exerts an independent effect to improve insulin sensitivity and glucose tolerance in genetically obese animal models (Cawthorne et al 1984). All of these effects are similar to those produced by exercise-training in Zucker rats and in man.

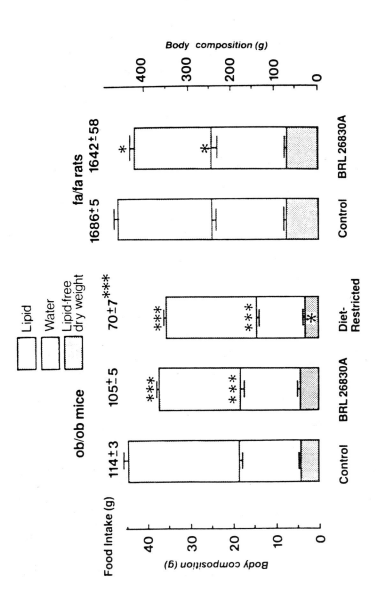

Figure 3. *Effects of BRL 26830A and diet restriction of body composition of ob/ob mice and fa/fa rats.* The mice (mean initial body weight 38 g) were dosed daily with water or BRL 26830A (10 mg/kg p.o.), or they were restricted to 60 per cent of the control food intake for 4 weeks. The rats (mean initial body weight 310 g) were dosed daily with water or BRL 26830A (1.9 mg/kg p.o.) for 12 weeks. $n=8$ (mice) or 6 (rats). Significance, relative to control values, is shown for food intake, final body weight, body lipid and lipid-free dry weight, which were measured as previously described. $*P<0.05$, $**P<0.001$.

Clinical studies have demonstrated that BRL 26830A was effective over 6 weeks in obese subjects, who were also adhering to a diet (Zed et al, 1985) but it was ineffective in refractory obese subjects (Chapman et al 1985). Connacher et al (1987) have recently shown that BRL 26830A produced a significantly greater weight loss than placebo over an 18 week period. Skin-fold and urinary N_2 excretion measurements were consistent with fat being the major component of the weight loss.

Acknowledgements

The originator of many of the ideas that led to the development of thermogenic agents in the treatment of obesity was Derek Miller, (Queen Elizabeth College, London), who died earlier this year. The author would like to dedicate this manuscript to him in appreciation of Derek's friendship and constant encouragement over many years.

References

1. Abraham RR, Densem JW, Davies P, Davie MWJ and Wynn V. The effects of triiodothyronine on energy expenditure, nitrogen balance and rates of weight and fat loss in obese patients during prolonged caloric restriction. Int J Obesity 1985, *9:* 433-442.

2. Arch JRS, Ainsworth AT, Cawthorne MA. Thermogenic and anorectic effects of ephedrine and congeners in mice and rats. Life Sciences 1982, *30:* 1817-1826.

3. Arch JRS, Ainsworth AT, Cawthorne MA, Piercy V, Sennitt MV, Thody VE, Wilson C and Wilson S. Atypical β-adrenoceptor on brown adipocytes as target for anti-obesity drugs. Nature 1984, *309:* 163-165.

4. Arch JRS, Brooks BJ, Thurlby PL and Wilson S. Sympathetic and hormonal regulation of brown adipose tissue thermogenesis. Biochem Soc Trans 1986, *14:* 230-233.

5. Arch JRS, Piercy V, Thurlby PL, Wilson C and Wilson S. Recent Advances in Obesity Research V (in press).

6. Boroumand M and Miller DS. An automated apparatus for measuring daily energy expenditure in laboratory animals. Proc Nutr Soc 1977, *36:* 14A.

7. Cawthorne MA, Carroll MJ, Levy AL, Lister CA, Sennitt MV, Smith SA and Young P. Effects of novel β-adrenoceptor agonists on carbohydrate metabolism: relevance for the treatment of non-insulin dependent diabetes. Int J Obesity 1984, 8 (Suppl 1) 93-102.

8. Chapman BJ, Farquhar D, Galloway S, Simpson GK and Munro JF. The effects of BRL 26830A, a new β-adrenoceptor agonist in refractory obesity. Int J Obesity 1985, *9:* 230.

9. Connacher AA, Jung RT and Mitchell PEG. Int J Obesity (in press).

10. Dulloo AG and Miller DS. The thermogenic properties of ephedrine methylxanthine mixtures in animal studies. AM J Clin Nutr 1986a, *43:* 388-394.

11. Dulloo AG and Miller DS. The thermogenic properties of ephedrine methylxanthine mixtures in human studies. Int J Obesity 1986b, *10:* 467-482.

12. Hollands MA, Arch JRS and Cawthorne MA. A simple apparatus for comparative measurements of energy expenditure in human subjects: the thermic effect of caffeine. Am J Clin Nutr 1981, *34:* 2291-2294.

13. Malchow-Moller A, Larsen S, Hey H, Stokhold KH, Juhl E and Quaade F. Ephedrine as an anorectic: the study of the "Elsinore pill". Int J Obesity 1981, *5:* 183-187.

14. Meier MK, Alig L, Burgi-Saville ME and Muller M. Phenethanolamine derivatives with calorigenic and anti-diabetic qualities. Int J Obesity 1984, 8 *(Suppl 1):* 215-226.

15. Miller DS in Proceedings of 2nd Conference on Regulation of Energy Balance (1974).

16. Miller DS and Stock MJ. A rapid method for the estimation of thermic energy in rats. Proc Nutr Soc 1969, *28:* 70A.

17. Pasquali R, Baraldi G, Gesari MP, Melchionda N, Zamboni M, Stafanini C, Raitano G. A controlled trial using ephedrine in the treatment of obesity. Int J Obesity 1985, *9:* 93-98.

18. Pasquali R, Cesari MP, Melchionda N, Stefanini C, Raitano A and Labo G. Does ephedrine promote weight loss in low-energy-adapted obese women? Int J Obesity 1987, *11:* 163-168.

19. Scoville BA. Obesity in Perspective 1974, 44-443.

20. Wellman PJ and Marmon MM. Synergism between caffeine and di-phenylpropanolamine on brown adipose tissue thermogenesis in the adult rat. Pharmacol Biochem Behav 1985, *22:* 781-785.

21. Wilson KL, Smith SA and Cawthorne MA. Comparative effects of voluntary exercise and caloric restriction of body composition and glucose tolerance in Zucher (fa/fa) rats. Int J Obesity 1984, *8:* 381.

22. Yen TT, McKee MM and Stamm NB. Thermogenesis and Weight Control. Int J Obesity 1984, *8 (Suppl 1):* 65-78.

23. Zed CA, Harris GS, Harrison PJ and Robb GH. Anti-obesity activity of a novel β-adrenoceptor agonist (BRL 26830A) in diet-restricted obese subjects. Int J Obesity 1985, *9:* 231.

Discussion

James: Could I just ask what happened to the anorectic drugs? Why the current interest in thermogenic drugs?

Cawthorne: There are two problems with the traditional anorectic drugs. Firstly their structural relationship with amphetamine and their potential for addiction and, secondly, the rate of weight loss which can be achieved was deemed by the FDA to be insignificant. It is anticipated that thermogenic drugs can do better.

Marks: Have you any idea how they actually work? Do thermogenic drugs increase lipolysis in fat liberating more fatty acids or do you think they actually increase metabolism within the adipolyte?

Cawthorne: In terms of mechanism of action I can only refer to the work with rodents and certainly, in them, there is increased metabolism in brown adipose tissue.

Marks: Most fat is not in brown adipose tissue, so do you get a rise in free fatty acids or in B-hydroxybutyrate or is there no discernible change in metabolites.

Cawthorne: Acutely you get a rise in free fatty acids which then disappears after chronic treatment. This does not necessarily mean lipolysis has stopped rather that there is an adaptation in brown adipose tissue enabling it to take up the free fatty acids as they are produced.

SOCIAL AND PSYCHOPATHOLOGICAL ASPECTS OF OBESITY

A H Crisp

Professor of Psychiatry
St George's Hospital Medical School, London

Introduction

The psychopathology of obesity is at least as complex and elusive as the biochemistry. Gorging and obesity itself are natural. In the past, survival in seasons of hardship was related to the body's capacity for consuming and storing excess. It is restrained eating that is the artefact and even a few days abstinence can unleash bulimia, as the obese know well.

Epidemiology of Obesity

Obesity is known to be related to age, gender and social class. The relationship with age and the association with gender are familiar. Many more females are obese than males which immediately implicates social and pscyhological as well as biological issues relating to gender roles and reproduction. The higher growth rate that characterises the female itself relates to obesity. The relationship with social class - obesity being more common in social classes IV and V (Silverstone, 1968) is probably still true today.

Cultural Influences

Those who have visited Japan or China recently will have noticed the relationship between the influx of the Western 'junk food' industry and massive obesity in children and adolescents in whom it was once very rare. This has doubtless been compounded by the social engineering in China of one child families.

Growth Rate

Obesity, certainly in the female, is clearly related to growth rate (Crisp et al, 1970). The more rapidly growth occurs through childhood, the more likely there is to be obesity before and after puberty. Puberty as an intervening factor does not seem to influence the association except tha partially reactive disorders such as anorexia nervosa and bulimia nervosa can occasionally erupt in the obese adolescent. Perhaps the shorter lifespan of the obese is programmed in that way.

Birth Order

Our data showed that obesity, defined as more than one standard deviation above the population mean, was significantly greater at 15 years of age in families where the proband was an only child, inevitably the first born, that survived to 15. This invites consideration of the psychopathology of the family with an only child. Otherwise obesity was commonest in the youngest which accords with what we know about multiparous women producing heavier babies as parity ascends probably related in turn to increasing maternal weight and the increasing capacity of her uterus.

Mood and Obesity

In the late 1960's we studied a South West London suburban population aged 40 - 65 years and found that obesity was correlated with low levels of anxiety in both males and females and also low levels of depression in males. This finding refers to the total number of obese, not the sub-population that actually complains of obesity. Considered overall, those aged 40 and over were significantly less dysphoric, even the females, than their non-obese counterparts. We then went on to study another population around a Cotswold market town, ranging from 17 - 70 years. The findings were upheld in respect of the population aged 40 and older and even in the males during the first half of life, but not in the females. With females, obesity in the younger age range was associated with dysphoria. Combining the data from the two studies the inescapable conclusion was that being thin was positively correlated with anxiety.

Furthermore, within that population, smoking tobacco was associated not only with being thin, but also with being anxious. The same applied to alcohol consumption Taking those who consumed large quantities of alcohol and also smoked tobacco there was a cluster of very thin middle-aged females who were also probably a population of chronic anorectics. So these data suggest significant relationships between mood, certain addictive behaviours and the state of obesity (Crisp, 1986).

Body Image

In the clinic population a striking feature has always been the predominance of female patients. This introduces a complicating psychological variable in any discussion of obesity because it reflects the fact that the obese female complains whereas the obese male, on the whole, does not. The female obese person's complaint relates to her dysmorphophobia.

In order to understand the background to this I refer to another survey we undertook (Crisp, 1985) of several thousand schoolgirls aged 12 - 19 years. Pubertal growth is largely finished by the age of 16 and then there is a rise in fatness followed by a reduction in fatness in the next year in this snapshot study (Figure 1). Two-thirds of the 18 year old schoolgirls said they would like to be a weight which was of anorectic (anorexia nervosa) proportions. They differed from anorectics in that they were not actually that weight. This dysmorphophobic propensity is one that a large proportion of females carry through into adult life and drives some of the obese amongst them to obesity clinics complaining bitterly and desperately that they are overweight.

The dysmorphophobia of the female is probably related to the construction of her gender role, conflict about it, and her adoption or rejection of her pubertally-driven sexuality. The male tackles his similar problems in ways that are less likely to involve obesity.

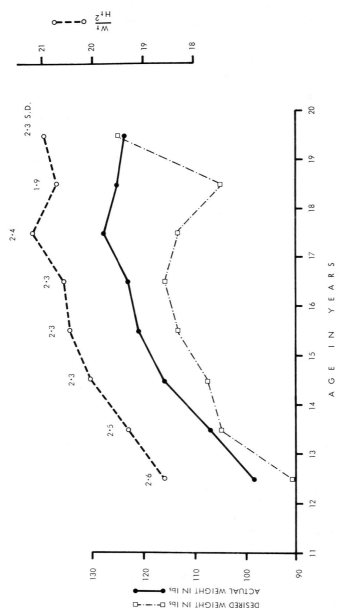

Figure 1: Mean "fatness" (measured height/weight) in a female adolescent school and college population (2,000 subjects). The increased "fatness" in the 17-18 year-olds could be based in selection factors (e.g. social class) for continued education at this period. However, the decline in "fatness" in the 18-19 year-olds probably relates more directly within the same population. One interpretation of the data is that as growth comes to a halt around 15-17 years, residual earlier adolescent binging persists, but within two years has subsided or been curbed by increasing dietary control associated with decrease in the desired weight. The desire to be slimmer is probably at its peak around this period especially in those who are on the plump side and have grown rapidly (Crisp, 1970), and the mean age of onset of anorexia nervosa itself is 17½ years.

31

Sexual Behaviour

In the clinic one is often dealing with massive obesity - 75% or more above the mean weight of a matched population. Such massive obesity is associated not only with general inertia in adolescents and in adults, which in itself can be important psychologically as a protective and defensive strategy and which then serves to perpetuate the obesity, but also specifically with sexual inactivity. An obese population is significantly less sexually active than it was pre-morbidly and less sexually active than matched controls (Crisp, 1967).

We studied the protective function of obesity in more detail (Crisp et al, 1977) in a population of massively obese female patients who experienced enforced rapid loss of weight (mean 40kg) following jejuno-ileal bypass surgery. This, we had expected, would provide us with an excellent population in which to study the psychological impact of weight loss in the absence of dieting. In fact, the weight loss was almost entirely due to post-operative enforced reduction of food intake and retention. As the women lost very large amounts of weight they became more generally active, more sexually active, more assertive and relationships, including marriages, were sometimes unexpectedly severed. Safe in the knowledge that they could not gain weight these women now began to prefer an image fatter than they actually were, emphasising the relationship of dysmorphophobia with problems about control.

Thus the inertia of massive obesity can be powerfully psychologically protective in the ways I have just suggested and may be one explanation for our findings of low anxiety in the obese.

Psychoanalytic Interpretation of Obesity

Feeding behaviour from birth becomes intimately bound up in additional human significance. The psychoanalysts have been perspicacious enough to portray a picture that we should not ignore. The nature of the bond with the mother is central with its sexual, physically intimate aspects later capable of being inflamed by incest, puberty and oedipal feeling. Compliant overeating and consequent obesity in childhood can be evidence of conflict avoidance behaviour in an excessively nurturing, fundamentally ambivalent mother, whose love is conditional as she unwittingly propels her child rapidly into the adult sexual world which she knows less about.

Food and 'junk' food is commonly used for reward and punishment in childhood and becomes significantly more complex as social and biological currency once adolescence has erupted.

Natural History of Obesity: An Illustrative Case History

There remains a lot to learn about the psychopathology of obesity by studying its natural history, a rather difficult process given the propensity for denial which obese people display.

This is the story of Lucy (Crisp, 1986). She was born the youngest child, weighing 3kg, of an unwanted pregnancy but was accommodated by her mother in an effort to restore an ailing marriage.

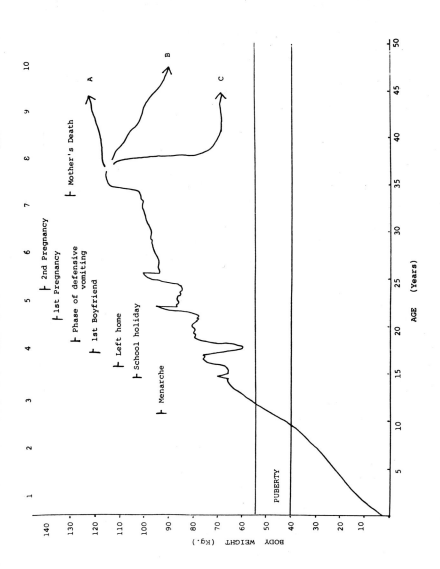

Figure 2: The development of massive obesity in an illustrative case, 'Lucy', with three possible outcomes, A, B or C.

Figure 2 illustrates her progress as she gained weight very rapidly throughout childhood. She entered early into puberty and adolescence by which time she was being teased and was socially withdrawn and her father had deserted the family. At the age of 15 she went away on her first school holiday. She came back weighing an extra 4kg, had missed a menstural period and her mother, who also conceived her first child out of wedlock and had been guiltridden about it ever since, believed her daughter to be pregnant. Lucy then dieted and her next period was a heavy one believed thereafter by her mother to have been an abortion.

At the age of 16 the patient leaves home and goes to live in London and attends a secretarial course. Her reaction to the separation in the first three months is to eat excessively. She then realises she must control her life and embarks on her first serious dieting and manages to reduce to 60kg. She has her first sexual experience apart from some previous incestuous behaviour with her father and her older brother before they left and deserted the home respectively. The relationship is not very satisfactory and she is abandoned by her boyfriend and goes back home to live and binges until she weighs 80kg.

By now the only way she can contain her weight is by secret vomiting which she does for the next four years. During this time she enters into another unsatisfactory relationship, becomes pregnant on her honeymoon and whilst pregnant gains 15kg, the pregnancy representing a licence to eat, being no longer associated with sexuality but with maternity. She is then left with her baby, 6kg heavier than she was before the pregnancy. She loses a little weight, is almost enticed into an affair with the man next door, resists and instead has another child by her husband and again increases massively in weight to 90kg.

Over the next 10 years she leads a fairly solitary life. She is insecure and dysphoric, obese, and still under the age of 40. But to the outside observer she keeps up the appearance of being a competent person. Her mother, whom she has more or less broken away from and ignored, then dies and she personally feels to blame. As part of the reparation she eats excessively and gains another 10kg to reach 110kg. We might leave Lucy at this point, grossly obese and sadly but compliantly reconciled to her fate (Course A). However, let us be optimistically interventionist and consider two other possibilities.

(Course B): She begins to feel that she can make something of her life. She takes her general practitioner's advice and attends the evening slimming clinic run by his community nurse. The community nurse seems to care. She talks to the group frankly about relevant aspects of her life and enables them to do the same and for the first time in her life Lucy feels part of the family. She slowly and steadily loses weight. As time goes by she is destined to become increasingly confident and assertive. She relates better to her children. She stays with her husband and organises their lives together in an effective way whereas previously she had dominated him in an hysterical fashion as part of her need to protect her own excessive vulnerability. Lucy's weight will plateau around 75kg in later life and she will be content.

(Course C): She is referred to the physician at the local district general hospital who advises a surgical approach which she accepts. Following ileojejunal bypass she loses 43kg over the next 6 months before her weight plateaus at just below 70kg. This is less than she has ever weighed since the age of 17 years. She feels as she did at that time when she had her first real boyfriend, and this time she feels more confident that she will not increase in weight and get fatter. Clinical complications arise as a result of the malabsorption and are going to trouble her in the future, but despite the diarrhoea and vomiting she gets if she eats unwisely, she now feels a different person and is confronted by the need to cope with her changed state. She finds that once again she is attracted to men, becomes involved in an affair and leaves her husband. She settles down in this new relationship taking her two children and they thrive. Her erstwhile husband becomes depressed.

The Outcome of Obesity: An Illustrative Case History

This is Sheila's story (Crisp and Stonehill, 1970), Sheila who is surely too emphatically programmed to be obese to ever avoid it unless, of course, she became anorectic. She comes from a modest home in the country, born the middle child of 5 into a family with a reputation for having a cupboard full of skeletons. Because of overcrowding she is sent at the age of 13 years to live with her grandmother.

Her grandmother is the person in this family who promotes the importance of food and of sitting round the table as the emblem of family unity and evidence of care. The move coincides with Sheila's early adolescence and she begins to enact the family psychopathology in a very modest way by staying out late and evokes great concern in the grandmother who at that point dies from a cerebral haemorrhage.

The family blame Sheila whose remorse for misbehaving resonates with this and she enters but never escapes from the bereavement process by beginning reparatively to overeat. She attempts to re-establish the bond in this pathological way so that by the age of 20 she weighs 20 stone. By then she has become inert and socially withdrawn. The obesity is the means by which she remains linked in to the family value system and is ultimately forgiven. Her weight creeps up to 25 stone at which point she eventually attracts medical attention and was referred to me.

We attempted to unravel the psychopathological elements of her story in hospital with the intention of treating her and her family. She was to receive dietary restriction and family and individual psychotherapy. She stayed in hospital for a year, from the age of 28 to 29, and we studied her intensively, measuring her activity during the day with pedometer and also her sleep patterns because we were interested in the relationship of diet, weight and sleep (Crisp and Stonehill, 1970).

She ate a 500 calorie diet for a whole year and she lost weight from 24 to 16 stones. The parents eluded us - they would not attend. They saw the threat, the potential for destabilising the situation psychologically and socially. The psychotherapy which sustained Sheila during that weight loss was actually aimed at grief work, enabling her to examine the origins of her behaviour such that she was able to work through her loss and resolve her grief. We were ultimately able to record that, whilst our patient lost her 8 stones, the remainder of the family gained an almost equivalent amount, including a new young sister-in-law incorporated into the family to replace the patient.

Our patient developed an active social life, still fairly obese but not psychogically or socially crippled, with a boyfriend, and the only price she paid was to be distanced from the family. Because she had challenged the family value system she was now on her own.Several outcomes were perhaps possible at this stage.She might theorectically, have developed bulimia nervosa. Alternatively, she might have developed a total avoidance response and anorexia nervosa. She did neither but remained obese, which was constitutionally a more likely outcome, but continued to curb further weight gain and no longer complained.

These two case histories illustrate the way in which loss can trigger massive weight gain. In like vein I have seen late onset diabetics have their disorder precipitated by overeating in response to the loss of a spouse. In order to control the condition it is necessary to tackle the psychopathology as well as the diabetes. Diet alone is often unsuccessful.

Summary

In summary, obesity and personality come to be closely related within an individual's constitution. The obesity is as resistant and as malleable to fundamental change as is the personality. Obesity may be protective against dysphoria and against potentially conflict-laden relationships because of its psychobiological nature.

Obesity is related to social class, gender and birth order in ways that defy simple explanations but which invite biological and psychosocial considerations. It relates to nurturing influences in childhood and psychopathologically it is vastly complicated by puberty which can precipitate massive obesity, bulimia nervosa or anorexia nervosa. The natural history of its evolution invites careful clinical study as a preamble to further clinical understanding.

References

1. Silverstone, JT. Psychosocial aspects of obesity. Proceedings of the Royal Society of Medicine 1968; *61:* 371.

2. Crisp AJ, Douglas JWB, Ross JM and Stonehill E. Some developmental aspects of disorders of weight. Journal of Psychosomatic Research 1970; *14:* 313-320.

3. Crisp AH. Some psychopathological aspects of obesity. In: Lacey JH and Sturgeon DA (Eds) Proceedings of the 15th European Conference on Psychosomatic Research. London, John Libbey, 1986: 129 - 128.

4. Crisp AH. Regulation of the self in adolescence with particular reference to anorexia nervosa. Transactions of the Medical Society, London, 1985; *100:* 67-74.

5. Crisp AH. The possible significance of some behavioural correlates of weight and carbohydrate intake. Journal of Psychosomatic Research 1967; *11:* 117-131.

6. Crisp AH, Kalucy RS, Pilkington TRE and Gazet JC. Some psychosocial consequences of ileojejunal bypass surgery. American Journal of Clinical Nutrition 1977; *30:* 109-120.

7. Crisp AH and Stonehill E. Treatment of obesity with special reference to seven severely obese patients. Journal of Psychosomatic Research 1970; *14:* 327-345.

DISCUSSION

Audience: Much research has been designed to answer the question of whether the high insulin secretion seen in obese people can be reproduced in normal people by overfeeding and therefore is a consequence of obesity rather than an aetiological factor. Do you think the same is true of GIP?

Marks: I believe that it is both aetiologically important and inducable i.e. secondary. In a genuine interrelated situation neither takes precedence. Both the hyperphagia and the hyperinsulinaemia/hypergipaemia which occur in the ob/ob obese mouse and in some humans are genetically determined. The hypergipaemia probably comes first in some instances. When obese mice are starved for 24 hours their plasma GIP levels certainly fall but not to such low levels as in the thin mouse. We have not been able to carry out experiments on human beings for long enough to see what happens to obese subjects who achieve normal weight on a normal diet and then to determine whether their GIP levels do indeed fall to normal levels. I believe that ordinarily GIP secretion and obesity is a linked phenomenon. That is, if you have hyperphagia without increased GIP and insulin secretion you do not become fat. You would not then deposit fat in your adipose tissues, you would instead burn it off. This is why I am interested to know the site at which the thermogenic drugs are postulated to exert their effect.

James: But underlying all this you would maintain that insulin is the mediator for the process?

Marks: Yes.

Lean: The stories are not imcompatible but it is quite difficult to tie the GIP story into the energetic equation which ultimately produces and maintains obesity. To return to the brown adipose tissue question, as a postulated site of action for thermogenic drugs, this is important if only as an analogy. Animal brown adipose tissue is very important in the response to feeding and although not intrinsically abnormal it does not respond in the normal way in the congenitally obese animal. In humans the tissue has the same biochemical function but its thermogenic capacity is very different in adults. It is present as a distinct tissue in foetal life and infancy and remains distinct biochemically in adults but is not quantitatively extensive enough to account for obesity.

Audience: It may well be that if two groups of people overeat those with the genetic predisposition or the higher GIP will become obese, but you still have to overeat for it to become manifest. So even if people have higher levels of GIP that does not explain why they overeat.

Marks: I did not suggest GIP causes hyperphagia. We start off with hyperphagia. The amount of energy that is expended depends on the amount of energy that is readily available to be burnt off. If you increase energy expenditure at the expense of intake you will lose weight which is why a thermogenic drug may work. We already have endogenous thermogenic hormones e.g. thyroxine and adrenaline. On the other hand you cannot get fat without insulin. GIP is designed to ensure that insulin is available when a meal is eaten and together they ensure that fat is taken up by adipose tissues.

Audience: Did you not say that people with high levels of GIP, albeit genetically determined, are obese because they eat more as a result of this?

James: No, what is being said is that the reason for eating more is unknown but that if people eat more then it is the GIP that actually selectively stimulates insulin which in turn programmes the fuel disposal so that it tends to be deposited more readily rather than invoking thermogenesis.

Cawthorne: It is not actually insulin level that determines the deposition of fat but rather the relative sensitivities and resistences of the tissues that determines whether thermogenesis or storage takes place.

Audience: Is there a GIP antagonist and can you raise antibodies to it?

Marks: GIP antibodies are very difficult to produce. There are no specific GIP antagonists except somatostatin. We plan to do some immunoneutralisation studies with GIP when we have purified our existing stocks of sheep anti-GIP but if you are using rabbits to raise the anti-GIP it is quite difficult to produce enough for long term immunoneutralisation.

James: In other words it is incredibly difficult to elucidate the specific mechanisms of GIP. It is probably the subtleties of energetics that are going to be the key. You appear to be looking at very small differences between people so that if there is some amplification system whereby you can look not at the 1% or 2% differences that make a person fat or thin but actually examine the process that is responsible then you may have a better discriminator. Perhaps the GIP story is such a process. Dr Lean, would you accept the proposition that some people can eat a great deal and just burn it off?

Lean: I think the slides Dr Cawthorne showed of enormous differences in food intake in people of the same weight have to be taken with a pinch of salt! Any measurement of food intake in the context of obesity or weight gain is highly suspect. There is a variation in food intake but it is not nearly as great as the old literature lead us to believe.

Cawthorne: I agree that it is not as great as the old literature led us to believe but, at the same time, it is true to say that when weight, sex and occupation are controlled there is still a variability which is sufficient to account for obesity.

James: In some way people do vary their food intake and in a controlled way. What you were looking at was not at the features of the control itself but at what the process was whereby one might achieve balance. We have heard about insulin and GIP - what about the autonomic system and brown fat?

Lean: Brown fat is the only tissue with a specific thermogenic mechanism, and this is under sympathetic, noradrenergic control. What is interesting is that brown fat persist into adulthood, and although inactive, it can be stimulated. Classically this is seen in the presence of phaeochromocytoma under massive noradrenaline stimulation at which time the measured capacity for thermogenesis and uncoupled respiration in the adipose tissue is dramatically increased. Again the question of thermogenic drugs is raised because if it is possible to selectively stimulate adipose tissue in this way it might be very useful therapeutically.

Cawthorne: Brown fat has probably led us astray in terms of human obesity. It is quantitatively much more important in rodents than in man. Muscle is quantitatively the major thermogenic tissue in man. In animals, brown adipose tissue has been useful for typing receptor action and fortuitously it would seem that in both muscle and white adipose tissue the receptors involved in lipolysis and thermogenesis are similar to the brown fat receptor.

Audience: How important do you think the thermogenic effect of exercise is?

Lean: You have to work very hard to generate enough calories to make a significant deficit. Of more interest is whether people respond differentially to exercise. It is a useful adjunct to other forms of therapy, but does not explain the aetiology of obesity. The obese do not expend less energy during exercise than lean people.

Cawthorne: It is not just the immediate cost of the exercise which should be considered but also the alterations over long periods of post-exercise time in basal metabolic rate.

James: Are you implying that it puts it up?

Cawthorn: Yes.

James: Summary of morning discussion:-
We do not really know what is going on in terms of the mechanisms

underlying the development of obesity and the two axes have to be considered viz. food intake and energy expenditure. Some believe the problem to be related to energy expenditure whilst others remain convinced there is also an excessive intake. In therapy there is now increasing interest in thermogenic compounds but as Professor Crisp has reminded us, when we take on those who come to clinics 'complaining' of obesity we have a real challenge to unearth all the interactions between their social and psychological problems and the metabolic factors which make them prone to obesity.

OVERVIEW: EXPECTATIONS OF TREATMENT

J A Garrow

Rank Professor of Human Nutrition
Medical College of St Bartholomew's Hospital, London

Introduction

Obese people can expect to lose weight at the rate of 1 or 2 pounds a week and to maintain that weight loss if they are careful. The severely obese who lose a lot of weight can expect their breathlessness, blood pressure and congestive cardiac failure to improve as also their joint pain, hypercholesterolaemia and type II diabetes. The advantages of weight loss to those with infertility or those preparing for elective surgery have not been so clearly demonstrated but would also seem to be reasonable goals. What is unreasonable is to expect to lose 4 to 7 pounds a week and to anticipate rejuvenation and miraculous improvements in failing marital relationships. Social success, depression and tiredness may or may not improve with weight loss.

Epidemiological Evidence for Benefits of Treatment

There is very good evidence taken from the experience of the Metropolitan Life Insurance Company that weight loss improves expectation of life. Those who were 25% overweight had an excess mortality of 39% but among 1300 people who lost weight mortality fell to a mere 11%. In those who were 35% overweight a 79% excess mortality was recorded which fell to only 9% among the 400 who lost weight. These are not ideal statistics but they do suggest that the excess mortality associated with obesity is reversible to some extent by weight loss.

The Framingham data show that it is not just the survival index which is affected by weight changes but also the risk factors of raised cholestrol, blood pressure, glucose and uric acid levels.

Patient's Expectations of Treatment

In a survey (Pacy, 1987) of the attitudes of those attending the Northwick Park Hospital for weight reduction, shortness of breath was the commonest reason followed by a desire to improve appearance in both sexes. Pain in weight bearing joints, hypertension and losing weight in preparation for gallstone, hip or knee surgery were surprisingly infrequent reasons given for wanting to lose weight.

The next question concerns the rate at which people expect to reduce. Munro (Ford et al, 1977) asked patients this and found that 32% thought that 1 or 2 pounds per week was reasonable, 40% expected to lose 2 - 4 pounds and 28% expected more than 4 pounds weight loss per week. These are quite unreasonable expectations which originate from the marketing claims of the various companies who manufacture diets. Reduction of 16 - 20 pounds per month is a frequently promoted claim. This being the case it is rather surprising that more patients do not actually believe it.

This is not to deny that such rates of weight loss are possible but they are neither frequently achieved nor desirable. Consider briefly what a weight loss of 4 - 7 pounds per week actually signifies. In a 70 kilogram man nearly two thirds of his body weight consists of water, 12 kilograms is protein and 12 kilograms is fat.

If a 10% increase in body weight was equally distributed across all compartments and a 10% decrease similarly constituted then weight loss would be a good index of treating obesity. If, on the other hand, obesity was reflected in increases only in the fat component then weight gain and loss would simply reflect changes in fat content. Unfortunately the relationship between body fat and body weight is much more complicated.

By weighing and measuring body fat in many patients at Northwick Park Hospital we found that more than 90% of the variation in body weight was indeed accounted for by variation in body fat.

For every kilogram of fat gained a 1.27 kilograms increase in weight was recorded. In other words the weight which people gain is 3/4 fat and 1/4 lean. Therefore, when they are losing weight, what they need to do is to lose weight which is also 3/4 fat and 1/4 lean. In the example of the 70 kilogram man, if he were to double his fat mass he would put on 12 kilograms of fat plus an extra 4 kilograms composed of 3 kilograms water and 1 kilogram protein.

During starvation the weight loss is not 3/4 fat and 1/4 lean but 50/50 fat and lean which means that an obese person can reduce to a normal weight without achieving normal body composition.

In order to achieve nomal body composition then every kilogram lost ought to contain 3/4 fat and 1/4 fat free mass. Using rather convenient arithmetic and assuming the energy supplied by fat is 9 cal per gm then the caloric distribution of the fat compartment is 6750 and of the fat free mass is about 250 adding up to a total of 7000 calories per kg. Therefore to lose 1 kilogram or 2.25 pounds per week there needs to be an energy deficit of 7000 calories a week or 1000 calories a day. The inherent fallacy of the claim that it is possible to lose 15 pounds per week (7kg) on a VLCD now becomes apparent as this represents an energy deficit of 49,000 calories which is greater than a person's total energy expenditure.

Very frequently patients are too optimistic about the rate of weight loss and when these expectations, which are, indeed, supported by manufacturers' advertisements, are not fulfilled, they then conclude they have a metabolic defect and they either become discouraged or turn up at an obesity clinic demanding an investigation.

There are also those who are too pessimistic in their expectations of weight loss. Astwood, the President of the American Endocrine Society, for example, stated categorically in his presidential address that "obesity is an inherited disorder due to a genetically determined defect in an enzyme," implying that people who are fat are born fat and nothing can be done about it! Bolden (1975) concludes in a similarly nihilistic vein that weight reduction programmes for the average patient in general practice are worthless.

Given these attitudes refractory obesity becomes a self-fulfilling diagnosis. If you assure an obese patient that his obesity is due to a genetic defect and he cannot lose weight then he will not lose weight. But we can probably do better than that.

Expectation of Increased Output

To return to first principles, obesity occurs when energy input exceeds energy output and is stored as fat. If the situation can be reversed so that energy output exceeds input then obesity becomes treatable. There are, of course, those in whom it is not possible to decrease energy input because they will not diet but the more interesting problem concerns energy output. Are there, in fact, obese people in whom the total energy expenditure is so low, either initially or in response to a diet, that effectively they cannot lose weight? In my experience the answer is no.

On average, obese people have both higher resting metabolic rates and higher total energy expenditures than lean people and therefore there is really no reason why they should not lose weight, at least, as well or better than lean people. There is plenty of good evidence for this (Blaza and Garrow, 1983; Ravussin et al, 1982; Schutz and Jequier, 1986; Blair and Buskirk, 1987; Prentice et al, 1986).

Summary

So when you are asked why, if obese people are metabolically normal, they do not lose weight on a reducing diet the answer is that they do. Given the appropriate prison camp conditions where food intake is completely controlled they **will** lose weight but, albeit, at widely differing rates. Overall though, a reasonable expectation of weight loss is in the range of 1 to 2 pounds per week until a refractory state is reached. Accompanying the weight loss it is reasonable to expect a melioration of the conditions discussed at the beginning.

References

1. Blair D, Buskirk ER. Habitual daily energy expenditure and activity levels of lean and adult-onset and child-onset obese women. American Journal of Clinical Nutrition 1987; *45:* 540-550.

2. Blaza S, Garrow JS. Thermogenic response to temperature, exercise and food stimuli in lean and obese women, studied by 24 h direct calorimetry. British Journal of Nutrition 1983; *49:* 171-180.

3. Bolden KJ. Against the active treatment of obesity in general practice. Update 1975; *2:* 339-348.

4. Ford MJ, Scorgie RE, Munro JF. Anticiapated rate of weight loss during dieting. International Journal of Obesity 1977; *1:* 239-243.

5. Pacy PJ, Webster JD, Pearson M, Garrow JS. A cross-sectional cost/benefit audit in a hospital obesity clinic. Human Nutrition: Applied Nutrition 1987; *41A:* 38-46.

6. Prentice AM, Black AE, Coward WA, Davies HL, Goldberg GR, Murgatroyd PR, Ashford J, Sawyer M, and Whitehead RG. High levels of energy expenditure in obese women. British Medical Journal 1986; *292:* 983-987.

7. Ravussin E, Burnand B, Schutz Y, Jequier E. Twenty-four hour energy expenditure and resting metabolic rate in obese, moderately obese, and control subjects. American Journal of Clinical Nutrition 1982; *35:* 566-573.

8. Schutz Y, Jequier E. Energy expenditure. Lancet 1986; *i:* 101-102.

Discussion

James: Is it now possible to assess what a person's expected energy expenditure should be given their weight?

Garrow: You can do this but not accurately. We had an approximately 10% error in our calculations of resting metabolic rate which is 73% of total energy expenditure. What you can do if you have a patient who is not losing weight on an 800 calorie diet is to measure their resting metabolic rate which will give you a baseline. A handy rule of thumb for converting oxygen consumption is O_2 mls/min x 7 = cals/day. An 120 kg man would need to have an oxygen uptake of 177 mls/O_2/min in order to be in energy balance on an 800 calorie diet.

James: Knowing you have an error term is it unreasonable to arrive at an estimate for expected energy expenditure?

Garrow: The problem with estimates is that they are based on average figures which do not seem to apply to any individual patient. What is needed is to set a lower limit for energy expenditure by measuring their metabolic rate. Patients and their GPs believe they are metabolically abnormal, firstly, because they have unreasonable expectations of what a normal rate of weight loss should be and secondly, because they are bad at recalling what they have eaten so that what they believe to be an 800 calorie diet is erroneous. Ordinary silver top milk contains 400 calories per pint, so it is a simple and accurate way to monitor a diet. If you drink 2 pints of milk per day and do not lose weight write to me!

DRUGS AND DIET

Professor T Silverstone
Professor of Clinical Psychopharmacology
Medical Colleges of St Bartholomew's and the London Hospitals

Why are there fat people? Everybody knows how to lose weight - you eat less and you exercise more - so why has obesity not disappeared? Because it is not easy to keep to a diet. For one thing, people get hungry and hunger is a most unpleasant feeling. Thus, one way of helping people to keep to a lower calorie diet is to help them reduce their hunger pharmacologically and there are a number of drugs available for this purpose. Today I want to discuss whether appetite suppressant drugs really work, how they work and whether they have a place in management.

Do Appetite Suppressant Drugs Actually Suppress Appetite?

The introduction of amphetamine as an appetite suppressant was quite fortuitous. It was originally synthesized in the late 1920's as a synthetic variant of ephedrine. Shortly afterwards its anorectic properties were recognised and it was then prescribed worldwide for many years as an appetite suppressant in the treatment of obesity until it fell from favour for reasons which will become apparent later.

In assessing the efficacy of anorectic drugs, visual analogue scales are often used to quantify hunger. Degree of hunger is marked along a horizontal line 10cm long which acts like a hunger thermometer and enables the effects of different drugs to be compared with those of placebo. Using visual analogue scales to measure hunger we have shown that fenfluramine, a non-stimulant appetite suppressant, is a highly potent anorectic drug in the 80mg dose but not at the plasma levels achieved by 40mg. 50mg diethylpropion in a single dose has also proven to be a statistically significant appetite suppressant reducing hunger ratings by nearly 50%, but is rather shorter acting as its pharmacokinetics would suggest.

Do Appetite Suppressants Reduce Food Intake?

The way that we have looked at this over the years is by using an automated solid food dispenser which records each item of food taken over a set period of time, thereby producing a cumulative food intake record. Comparing 75mg diethylpropion and 60mg fenfluramine with placebo, both anorectic drugs caused a marked reduction in the amount of food that subjects ate during the course of 8 hours of unrestricted access to the feeding machine.

So these drugs **do** reduce appetite and they **do** reduce food intake in single dose, single day experiments in normal subjects but do they actually help obese people lose weight?

Do Drugs Help Obese People Lose Weight?

John Munro and his colleagues many years ago, compared a number of drugs in resistant obesity and showed that they all work, some rather better than others. Fenfluramine had a more persistant effect but amphetamine and dexamphetamine certainly helped patients lose weight and the inference is that they were working by helping patients keep to a low calorie diet. All patients were given the same diet but those on placebo did not seem to keep to it probably because they get hungry. Dietary compliance is enhanced by drugs because hunger is less insistent. So patients do find them helpful.

Margaret Ashwell did a very detailed survey of acceptability and preference for these drugs among "Which" reader dieters, asking them whether they were unhelpful, helpful or very helpful. The commonly available drugs were rated as being quite helpful, whereas methycellulose, which we in another context, have shown **not** to suppress appetite at all, was quite unhelpful in the few patients who had taken it. Diethylpropion and fenfluramine clustered around the "quite helpful" rating, so patients believe them to be helpful and they do seem to produce weight loss in properly controlled clinical trials.

Duration of Efficacy

The critics of anorectic drug treatment say that they work in the short term but they do not re-educate the patient to eat properly so their effect is limited. Drugs are effective for as long as they are taken which is all we can reasonably expect of them. But how long should you go on treating with drugs?

Munro has shown with fenfluramine that if you can achieve high enough plasma drug levels i.e. 200 ng per ml it is possible to show highly significant weight loss persisting over 20 weeks. With lower blood levels the effect rapidly wears off; this looks like a dose-response effect or more specifically, a plasma level response effect, with the high plasma level causing a much more effective and persistent loss of weight.

If you switch over from active drug to placebo when weight loss has plateaued then weight is immediately regained. This suggests that the drug must be doing something even when apparent weight loss has ceased. Clearly, the drugs are effective as long as they are taken, but we do not yet know for how long they should be taken. Currently running long terms trials should yield very interesting information, not only about how long the drugs work while they are being taken but also on the expected drop-out rate over 12 months.

Tolerance

The association of high plasma drug levels with persisting weight loss suggests that tolerance does not develop. Our own work brings out this point even more clearly comparing 3 groups of dieting patients. Group A took diethylpropion continuously for 4 month, Group B started on an active drug and then went on to placebo and Group C took placebo alternating monthly with active drug. Group A and B were initially indistinguishable but Group C on placebo lost 50% less weight. The next month the rate of weight loss fell in Group A, a feature that has often been attributed to tolerance, but also in Group C who had never had the drug before. If this fall-off truly reflected tolerance then Group C should have lost as much weight as Groups A and B in their first month.

It is, in fact, the compliance to dieting generally which declines over time, but there is still a drug effect because those who switched to placebo regained weight compared with those on active drug who merely stopped losing weight. There is no true pharmacological tolerance - what occurs is behavioural tolerance.

Dependence

Anorectic drugs do not cause physical dependence. If you stop taking them you do not get withdrawal symptoms; nor has psychological dependence been a major problem. Most patients who stop their appetite suppressants cope quite well. Some patients miss the lift they get from the stimulant type of drugs but fenfluramine does not have any stimulant action and **never** causes dependence, and diethylpropion only very rarely. So dependence really is not a serious problem.

Abuse

They can, however, be drugs of abuse. Abuse is defined as the self-administration of a substance in non-therapeutic doses for non-medical reasons, usually by non-patients. Amphetamine is still widely used (illegally) in this country as a "recreational drug" as are alcohol and cannabis. Amphetamine was withdrawn from the market for this reason but other substances of abuse such as glue have not been banned just because young adults sniff it. It seems to me to be quite irrational and inconsistent to take appetite suppressants out of the pharmacopeia simply because non-patients are abusing them.

Conclusions

I hope I have shown you that these drugs work - they reduce hunger, they reduce food intake, they thereby help people to stick to their diets and so help them to lose weight. The dangers associated with them have been exaggerated in my opinion. Fenfluramine is most useful for people who are anxious or perhaps overactive, and maybe diethylopropion or phentermine for the more anergic patient.

A whole new generation of appetite suppressant drugs are currently under review based on the principle of increasing 5HT neurotransmission. The dextro-isomer of fenfluromine is a selective 5HT releaser and there are two antidepressant drugs already either available or almost available, fluvoxamine and fluoxetine, both of which block the reuptake of 5HT and both of which have definite appetite suppressant properties.

These newer appetite suppressants can probably be used with a reasonable degree of confidence and safety. In general, anorectic drugs should only be used to help people to stick to a low calorie diet which, after all, is their sole purpose. Use should be largely restricted to those who are medically at risk i.e. those that are 30% above their ideal body weight and/or who suffer from the complications of obesity such as hypertension or type II diabetes. Here, these drugs have a real place in clinical management. The duration for which they should be prescribed is uncertain, but probably longer than previously thought. If may even be that with some patients they need to be taken for periods of years.

Silverstone - Discussion

Audience: Are there studies to monitor compliance?

Silverstone: We monitor plasma levels of drugs but that does not tell you directly about compliance.

Audience: What about compliance with diet?

Silverstone: Compliance is implied by evidence of weight loss. Diet diaries are not foolproof.

James: You have show that these drugs are anorectic but do any of them put up energy expenditure as well.

Silverstone: The stimulant ones can put up heart rate. I do not actually know the data about energy expenditure. Even if these drugs work in part by increasing energy expenditure their major impact is on energy intake.

WHY EVEN CONSIDER DRUGS?

J F Munro

Consultant Physician
Eastern General Hospital

and

S Stewart
SHO, Eastern General Hospital

In any condition drug therapy can only be justified if there are effective drugs available and if the condition itself is sufficiently serious to warrant treatment. The obese are potentially vulnerable to a wide variety of disadvantageous conditions. They have an increased liability to flat feet, varicose veins, varicose ulcers and arthritis of the weight-bearing joints. There is an increased incidence of various gynaecological malignancies, of gallstones and a worsening of the symptoms of hiatus hernia. Surgery becomes more difficult and complications such as incisional hernia are more frequent. In any condition causing breathlessness being overweight will increase the dyspnoea. There is an increased risk of hypertension, hyperlipidaemia and type II diabetes.

In addition to these physical problems which may require treatment some obese people are so distressed by their adiposity that this in itself is a justification for treatment. But this is a decision which is best taken by the patient. All the obese are in a sacrifice position and the choice they face is whether they are prepared to undergo the privations or changes in lifestyle necessary to bring about weight loss or whether to forego the advantages, as they perceive them, of weight loss and remain fat.

Treatment Options
General Considerations

The best treatment of all is prevention. Once obesity is established the next most effective form of treatment is self-control without recourse to dietitians, slimming organisations or the medical profession. Failing this, the next step is the development of a behavioural modification programme involving dietary restriction and exercise with or without group therapy. If this is not successful a more radical option may have to be considered. Drug therapy only becomes attractive if the alternatives are hazardous or ineffective.

Jejuno-Ileal Bypass Surgery

The concensus view not shared by everybody is that the successes of the

1960's and 1970's are the failure of the 1980's and that this is a procedure which should now be abandoned.

Gastric Surgery

There are a multiplicity of ways to exclude the stomach, the mere existence of so many procedures suggesting that none is ideal. No sooner have a few years experience been accumulated with a procedure such as horizontal gastroplasty, for example, than it is superceded by a newer technique such as vertical banding gastroplasty. Perhaps it should be reserved for those who have already lost substantial weight by another method but are unable to control weight regain. At best gastric surgery merely replaces the problems of obesity with those of a "small stomach syndrome".

Very Low Calorie Diets

The arguments both for and against VLCDs are passionate. Clearly, in comparing the efficacy of a 500 calorie diet with a 1000 calorie diet, if the difference in weight loss is in excess of a pound per week, it is at the expense of non-fat tissue. Possibly the principal advantage of a VLCD is that some people can adhere more easily to a completely liquid diet.

Kirschner's study on VLCD (Kirschner et al, 1987) is probably the most impressive so far published. These results need to be interpreted with caution. That 42% of their successfully slimmed group maintained their weight within 5kg over the ensuing 18 months is a remarkable achievement. However, it is important to appreciate that this represents no more than 10% of the subjects recruited into the programme. Another interesting feature of this study, and one which we have been able to reproduce, is that men do very much better than women. Furthermore, this holds every bit as true on conventional diets.

Jaw-Wiring

This is really a form of compulsory VLCD. As with other non-surgical forms of radical therapy weight regain during follow-up is very common.

Drug Therapy

It is thus, in the context of disappointing results from alternative treatment methods that we need to assess the contribution made by drugs. There are various different mechanisms whereby drugs can promote weight loss.

i) Enhancement of Thermogenesis

Thyroid hormones, given in pharmacological doses, are thermogenic but also catabolic and have no place in the treatment of obesity. A number of novel compounds are undergoing clinical evaluation. Dr Cawthorne has already described a number of these and it seems possible that BRL26830A will significantly accelerate the rate of weight loss in subjects already successfully reducing (Munro et al, 1987; Connacher et al, 1987).

ii) Reduction of Energy Intake

These drugs fall into two neuropharmacological groups - those working primarily on 5HT neurotransmitters such as fenfluramine, and others which work on the catecholaminergic systems within the brain and which have the disadvantages of being "stimulant."

iii)Impairment of Absorption

There is currently much interest in this class of compounds which work by producing nutrient malabsorption. Acarbose interferes with carbohydrate absorption and is being used in clinical trials in Germany in the management of diabetes. Tetrahydrolipstatin is another agent undergoing investigation, which mainly effects lipid asborption.

The division of drugs into these broad categories is an oversimplification. For example, agents which impair nutrient absorption may also indirectly impair food intake.

Indications for Drug Therapy
i)   General Considerations

The individual response to drug treatment is unpredicatable and is relatively unrelated to the choice of drug as many direct comparison studies show remarkable similarities in mean weight loss (Scoville, 1973).

Timing of treatment is a factor. Predictably, one would expect more weight loss can be attributed to drug treatment given when a patient first seeks medical assistance compared with withholding treatment until the weight loss caused by dietary restriction alone has plateaued.

With continuing drug treatment the extra weight loss will sooner or later stop though this does not necessarily imply that the drug is no longer producing an effect. Often weight reduction plateaus within weeks though with fenfluramine a mean weight reduction may continue for months (Steel et al, 1973).

The most important variable remains the individual patient. Even in subjects with refractory obesity the exceptional individual may lose vast amounts of weight (Steel et al, 1973). Possibly this relates to drug pharmacokinetics but the relationship is by no means straightforward. Possibly it relates to psychological factors such as whether or not an obese subject has a sympathetic partner which has been shown to influence the rate of reduction.

ii) Short Term Goals

Drug treatment can be most readily justified where there is an obvious need for short term weight loss such as to facilitate elective surgery or for some pressing social reason such as a wedding. In these circumstances the probability of subsequent weight regain may not be a valid contraindication to treatment. Nonetheless, the greatest drawback to drug treatment is that weight regain is the rule. Indeed, it has been suggested that subjects treated with a drug may in the long term finish up heavier than those managed without drug therapy

(Stunkard et al, 1980).

An alternative non-pharmacological approach involves the use of a nylon cord around the patient's waist. This technique was pioneered by Garrow who showed that in a substantial proportion of patients it minimised weight regain following dental splinting (Garrow and Gardiner, 1981). Similar results have been achieved using an adjustable waist cord following VLCD. It must be emphasised that the use of a waist cord is merely an adjunct to therapy not a solution in its own right.

iii) Long Term Therapy

There is anecdotal evidence that long term drug therapy can be used to prevent weight regain (Hudson, 1977; Enzie et al 1976; Craddock, 1987). Long term treatment is bedevilled by problems and prejudices. Possibly the fear of drug tolerance and drug addiction has been overstated but it cannot be totally discounted. Drugs have rarely been prescribed for lengthy time periods; the long term side effects have yet to be firmly established. Moreover subjects often become disillusioned once they have actually stopped losing weight whether or not substantial weight loss has already occurred.

It follows that the ideal anti-obesity agent will have not only a weight losing effect but some other clearly defined therapeutic benefit justifying long term use. Hypertension is one such indication and fenfluramine may have some hypotensive properties. Depression is another and a new generation of antidepressants, fluoxetine, fluvoxamine and femoxitine, are selective 5HT agonists which, theoretically, may possess the weight reducing properties of fenfluramine. A comparison of fluvoxamine with placebo (Abel et al, 1986) revealed no difference in weight loss but this can be considered to be a positive finding compared with the weight gain which accompanies tricyclics. The results with fluoxetine appear even more impressive (Ferguson, 1986).

An agent which selectively improves carbohydrate tolerance is a particularly attractive concept. Fenfluramine arguably does this (Doar et al, 1979). Metformin undoubtedly does it, the effect on weight being considerable when compared with chlorpropamide (Clarke and Duncan, 1968). A number of agents currently under evaluation - thermogenic drugs, drugs which interfere with nutrient absorption and possibly fluoxetine may also have beneficial effects on carbohydrate tolerance over and above that attributable to weight loss. If this is confirmed then their long term use in obese diabetics offers the opportunity to evaluate their long term safety and efficacy before their introduction as anti-obesity agents in the non-diabetic.

Drugs and Alternative Methods of Preventing Weight Gain

The short term indications for drug therapy could be more easily justified if a non-pharmacological method of preventing weight regain was available. The study by Stunkard (1980) has been widely quoted to imply that drug therapy negates the benefits of behaviour modification. It may well be, however, that the behaviour modification was given at the wrong time. There remains a need to formally assess the long term benefits of an intensive behaviour modification programme initiated when drug therapy is discontinued.

Summary

In conclusion, it is important to appreciate that weight loss itself is not the only prerequisite in the management of obesity. Sometimes it is more realistic to focus on preventing weight regain. Sometimes unrelated but important risk factors such as cigarette smoking are a greater health hazard than obesity. Sometimes the treatment of associated conditions, in particular hypertension and diabetes, or of the psychological implications of obesity are much more important therapeutic goals than weight reduction.

References

1. Abel CA, Farquhar DL, Galloway S McL, Steven Fiona, Philip AE, Munro JF. Placebo controlled double blind trial of fluvoxamine maleate in the obese. J Psychosomatic Res 1986; *30 (2):* 143-6.

2. Clarke BF, Duncan LJP. Comparison of chlorpropamide and metformin treatment on weight and blood glucose response of uncontrolled obese diabetics. Lancet 1968; *i:* 123-6.

3. Connacher AA, Jung RJ, Mitchell PEG. The antiobesity effect of BRL 26830A. Int J Obesity 1987; *11:* 307A.

4. Craddock D. The long term management of obesity by anorectic drugs: ten year follow up. Int. J. Obesity 1987; *11:* 305A.

5. Doar JWH, Thomson ME, Wilde CE, Sewell PFJ. The influence of fenfluramine on oral glucose tolerance tests, plasma sugar and insulin levels in newly diagnosed, late-onset diabetic patients. Curr Med Res & Opinion 1979; *6 (suppl 1):* 247-54.

6. Enzie G, Barotussop A, Machion E, Capaldi G. J. Int Med Res 1976; *4:* 305-18.

7. Ferguson JM. Fluoxetine induced weight loss in humans. In "Advances in the Biosciences - Disorders of Eating Behaviour: a Psychoneuroendocrine Approach" Eds. Ferrari E, Brambbilla F, Pergamon Press, Oxford, 1986; 313-18.

8. Garrow JS, Gardiner GT. Maintenance of weight loss in obese patients after jaw wiring. Br Med J 1981; *282:* 858-60.

9. Hudson KD. The anorectic and hypotensive effect of fenfluramine in obesity. JR Coll GP 1977; *27:* 497-501.

10. Kirschner MA, Schneider G, Ertel N, Gorman J. A very-low calorie formula diet program for control of major obesity: and 8-year experience. In "Recent Advances in Obesity Research: V" Proceedings of the 5th International Congress on Obesity. Eds Berr EM, Blondheim SH, Eliahou HE and Shafrir E. John Libbey, London, Paris 1987; 342-6.

11. Munro JF, Chapman BJ, Robb GH, Zed C. Clinical studies with thermogenic drugs. In "Recent Advances in Obesity Research: V" Proceedings of the 5th International Congress on Obesity Eds Berry EM, Blondheim SH, Eliahou HE, Shafrir E. John Libbey, London, Paris 1987; 155-9.

12. Munro JF, Douglas JG. The management of obesity. Human Nutrition: Clinical Nutrition 1983; *37C:* 1-19.

13. Scoville BA. Review of amphetamine-like drugs by the Food & Drug Administration. In "Obesity in Perspective - Proceedings of Fogarty Conference" Ed Bray GA

Washington, US Govt. 1973: 441-3.

14. Steel JM, Munro JF, Duncan LJP. A comparative trial of different regimens of fenfluramine and phentermine in obesity. Practitioner 1973; *221*: 232-6.

15. Stunkard AJ, Craighead LW, O'Brien R. Controlled trail of behavioural therapy, pharmacotherapy and their combination in the treatment of obesity. Lancet 1980; *2*: 1045-7.

LOW CALORIE DIETS: HOW LOW SHOULD YOU GO?

J Stordy

Senior Lecturer in Nutrition
University of Surrey, Guildford

DISCUSSION

Audience: Could anti-obesity drugs be used on patients who are obese because they are already taking drugs as is commonly seen in psychiatric patients on psychotropic preparations. Anti-depressants and tranquillisers often lead to weight gain and some patients stop taking them for this reason.

Silverstone: As far as the antidepressant weight gain is concerned the newer generation of antidepressants such as fluoxetine or fluvoxamine would be the treatment of choice. So instead of treating the antidepressant-induced weight gain with another drug it would be preferable to switch the patient to a non weight-increasing anti-depressant. As far as the neuroleptic-induced obesity is concerned this is a real problem. We did a survey of a clinic population of chronic schizophrenics who were receiving long term neuroleptic drugs and found that well over a third were clinically obese. They had a body mass index over 30 which really is unacceptably high when you think of the normal population prevalence of about 6-7%. Here anti-obesity drugs may have a role to play. We have just completed a double blind study of d-fenfluramine in such neuroleptically- induced obese patients and found that it was better than placebo.

Audience: Although we have heard about "follow-ups" of 2 years on patients who have lost weight, has any one followed up patients for 10 years?

Garrow: No, not many people have follow-ups of 10 years on all patients apart from anecdotal reports. I am a proponent of the waist cord for people who have lost a lot of weight because, provided they keep it on, they do not regain much weight. We have a mean follow-up of 3 years of those who had lost about 40 kilograms and the weight regained is about 9 kilograms. What you are asking for is what we all want, namely a properly followed-up complete series of people who have lost a lot of weight. GPs are in the best position to do these long term follow-ups because they are still in touch with the patients who soon lose contact with hospital clinics.

Munro: It is almost unethical when you have a patient who is regaining weight to just sit back and do nothing. So some form of further intervention is instituted and this then makes it very difficult to interpret the follow-up results. With surgery one can produce very good long term follow up results of seven years or so. The results for VLCD are somewhat ambiguous as it is often difficult to assess the number of patients who were initially treated.

Stordy: I think that is absolutely true. Hopefully Kirschner will be able to give very long term follow-ups on their large series of patients.

Audience: Has anybody done a study of a cocktail mixture of drugs such as an anorectic drug plus a thermogenic drug? I would have thought the ideal bedmates would have been fenfluramine and BRL 26830 in terms of side effects.

Munro: I am sure that particular combination has not been done, but fenfluramine and phentermine has. The idea of combining drugs fills me with horror, I would much rather see them used in series. If combinations are used and there are problems with side effects you have no idea which drug is at fault.

Audience: Regular exercise is claimed to be hazardous for the obese because it produces minor orthopaedic complaints but you can sit on an excercise bicycle and work out for 20 minutes a day without any danger. The benefits include improved diabetic control, lowering hypertension, effects on serum lipids and on osteoporosis and it has an anti-depressant effect as well. I would have liked Duphar to have invited an exercise physiologist to discuss the benefits of exercise in a dietary programme.

Garrow: All obese patients, indeed everyone, should be encouraged to exercise because it promotes physical fitness and also insulin sensitivity but the evidence for the effects of exercise on weight loss is very disappointing. The studies which show that exercise produces a prolonged increase in metabolic rate only hold true for Olympic class athletes. In our studies on the exercise levels achieved by ordinary civilians we have totally failed to reproduce the effect on prolonged increase in metabolic rate. With regard to the antidepressant effect a recently published study in which people were randomly assigned to exercise and non exercise treatments, failed to find a significant effect on mood. Obesity covers a wide spectrum of people and it is only a small proportion of these for whom an exercise programme can usefully be a large proportion of the treatment programme. However, in every treatment programme and indeed in ordinary non obese civilians, exercise should be promoted for its other beneficial effect.

Audience: We have looked at the effects of VLCD over a period of 4 weeks in patients with well established ischaemic heart disease and hypertension and find that there has been a dramatic improvement in symptoms and also in stress tests and in cardiac output. Furthermore, 50% of the hypertensive patients no longer required hypotensive medication. So it is not only weight loss but quality of life and other things that matter. I would also like to remind clinicians here that if they are considering VLCD it is most inappropriate to continue beta blockers and hypotensive therapy because of this observed effect.

Audience: Do VLCD actually achieve a reduction in fat tissue and spare the lean tissue?

Stordy: They achieve a substantial reduction in fat tissue, largely sparing lean tissue, particularly after the first two weeks. There is a period of adaptation when there is some loss of nitrogen mostly from the liver and the gut mucosa following which there is a continuing slight negative balance and loss of lean tissue. This is what you would expect because certain lean tissues are there in excessive quantities anyway.

Munro The biggest problem is that once again there is an enormous individual variation in nitrogen balance and that although this relates somewhat to size and gender, on the whole, people behave very differently when you subject them to considerable energy deficits.

Garrow: The question is a very good one - the key issue being whether the loss of lean tissue is excessive. I believe it is and the evidence is good for this. During starvation roughly 50% of the weight loss is lean tissue. On conventional diet, by which I mean 800+ calories the loss is about 25% and on VLCD it is somewhere in between. I agree entirely with John Munro's comments about why it is very difficult to answer this question absolutely. There is firstly, a large difference between individuals and secondly, the ratio of lean tissue loss to total weight loss changes with time. The longer you are on a diet, the relatively more efficient conservation becomes and obviously you cannot compare two diets at the same time. If you compare them sequentially quite complicated crossover experimental designs are necessary. Furthermore the ratio of lean tissue loss to total weight loss depends on the proceding diet so not only have you to do this crossover you also need a base line. My belief is that the loss of lean tissue on very low calorie diets is excessive.

James: The whole question of protein intake is intimately related to energy intake. The values which are recommended in the FAO report as being appropriate protein intakes pre-suppose energy balance. Much of the confusion about protein requirements that occurred in the early seventies related to energy overfeeding studies in America where the overfeeding reduced the supposed protein needs to inappropriately low levels. The evidence that we have so far, which is not very good, is that you need rather higher protein intakes if you are on lower energy diets and that may be part of the complication that we have got to try to cope with.

Munro: In looking at the old liquid diet experience the dangers were in people who were not very obese, or who were taking the preparation for a long time. In other words the degree of obesity is inversely proportional to the risk. Possibly the risks are greater in people who are using it cosmetically for short periods of time.

Stordy: Nitrogen requirements must be related to body size. Some of the individual variation in nitrogen equilibrium occurs because of body size differences and at least you should attempt to take account of this on VLCD.

Lean: Dr Stordy, can you enlarge on or defend your earlier suggestion that VLCD should be used intermittently? I worry that if used in a cyclical fashion for a slimming period followed by a re-feeding period, there may be cumulative effects on body composition and calcium status.

Stordy: I am sorry if that view got across at all because I certainly do not feel that VLCD should be used in a cyclical fashion. I consider they should be used to achieve a substantial energy deficit whether they are used as a sole regime or as a mixture with some additional food added as a sound nutritional basis for a low calorie diet. I do not agree with the recent article in the BMJ by Apfelbaum which suggested that they be used for a period of a month followed by a fuller diet and then possibly another month of VLCD because I agree that the adaptive process which is conserving nitrogren equilibrium and nutrients is being called into play more often and it is possible to get more severe negative nitrogen imbalance. Most of the long term studies have not used that type of approach. People have been consistently on a low energy intake of say 500 calories.

James: I am now getting a slightly different message. The very low calorie diets as you see them are best used for rather long periods of time. I am slightly concerned. There was a consensus at the Montreux Conference 2 years ago that VLCD should be used for only limited periods of time. Do you think that is now passé?

Stordy: There was never much published data to indicate this is the best way to use them. Most of the detailed studies are on prolonged continuous use of the dietary programmes so you cannot say that it is safer to use it 3 weeks on and 1 week off.

Garrow: This recommendation that a very low calorie diet should be used for 3 weeks at a time was really an administrative muddle. What happened was that since evidence was presented that no harm occurred during a period of 3 weeks the regulating agencies decided it could be recommended for 3 weeks. I agree with Dr Stordy that no one actually says the optimum way of using very low calorie diets is 3 weeks on and 1 week off.

James: Let us imagine that I am a dietician with a series of patients coming up in the next 12 months. Should I be assessing them, classifying them in specific ways, sending them out to Weight Watchers, giving them Cambridge Diets or Univite or should I sympathise and advocate a little less dietary fat and a little more protein intake?

Silverstone: Essentially what happens should be the patients decision. One should put very firmly to them that the option is their's, that dieting is a difficult and often unsuccessful endeavour and they should think very seriously before they wish to enter into it. Then having decided mutually that the strategy is to lose weight, the question of tactics is very much a matter of the individual needs in terms of degree of obesity, of support available and requirement for drugs. The type of diet is an equally important matter for the doctor, the dietitian, the 'professional' adviser and the patient to decide upon . Some people welcome the absolute limits set by liquid diets, others prefer to carry on in a more socially acceptable or conventional eating pattern. We cannot give you an answer you must use your clinical skills and professional empathy.

Marks: If you do not know the cause of obesity everything you do to treat it is purely empirical. You might or might not be successful but it can still only be symptomatic treatment. This idea that we know how to treat obesity is one of the things that has got to be dispelled. When we know what causes a disease - when we understand its pathology, then we have something that we can treat. Let us spend more money on research and less pretending that we know how to treat this condition.

Munro: Obviously I agree, but the parallel is to say let us not bother to treat hypertension or cancer unless there is a specific cause for it. To address the original question - there are a number of things one should ask at the time of initial referral. The first being to what does a person attribute their obesity. This is a very important question and one with many different answers. Secondly, why do they want to lose weight, because unless they have already considered this carefully they are not in a position to make a rational decision. Two further issues concern whether they have a realistic concept of the rate at which they can expect to lose weight and whether they have a realistic target weight. If I were to blame Weight Watchers for one thing, it would be for giving grossly obese people a totally unrealistic target weight. Finally, I feel we do not involve the patient sufficiently in the decision making process so that eventually they blame us for failure and we criticise them for failure. The way ahead must be to try and involve each one in the decisions made having provided them with the options.

Garrow: I can solve Professor James ' problems instantly. He says he is a dietitian with thousands of patients turning up so I suggest that the first thing he does is to classify them according to severity. The first step for any service, dietetic or public health, is to set up slimming groups in the community. If there are commercial ones that work - well and good - if there are not they should be set up as they are in Harrow Health District. You then have a filtering system, because in this way you can provide appropriate advice and support in these groups very inexpensively. You then need a back up system and the effective way of using hospital clinics is essentially to cope with people referred from community slimming groups which may be run by dietitians, commercial clubs or GPs. In this way the relatively rare and expensive hospital facilities could be used to greater effect than simply using them as the first port of call for everyone.

Audience: The role of the media is also very important in getting the right message across. A recent survey asked people where they got their nutrition and slimming information from. At the top of that list were newspapers and magazines and at the bottom were hospital dietitians and doctors. When those same people were asked who they believed the doctors came right at the top and newspapers and magazines came below. Another survey asked GPs where they got all their information about nutrition and it appears that they too get it from newspapers and magazines! I would like to see the media taking a much more responsible attitude to articles on slimming and nutrition. If you are contacted by journalists make certain that you spend time educating them and that you see what they write.

LIST OF DELEGATES

ABRAHAM R R
London

ADAMS J
London

ADDIS W D
Dorking

ALBAN DAVIES H
Cambridge

ANSTISS T
Hounslow

ARMON S
St Albans

ASHFORD J J
Southampton

ASHWELL M
London

BAWA H K
South End-on-Sea

BECKERS S R
Bridport

BEGLIN S
Oxford

BISHOP J M
Edenbridge

BORROWS A
Newport

BOWEN M
Nottingham

BOWNESS K J M
Brampton

BOWYER C
London

BROWN P J
London

BURLEY V
London

COUMAR A
London

CRICHLOW I
Harrow

CROWTHER P S
Windlesham

DAGGETT P R
Stafford

DAVIES R
London

DEBENHAM K A
Reading

DEVAKUMAR V C
Rossendale

De WET M
London

D'SOUZA J A G
Lancashire

EAKIN M A
Macclesfield

EELEY E
Oxford

ELLIS L J
Harrow

ENOCH B A
Manchester

ENSER M B
Bristol

EVANS E
London

FAIRBURN C G
Oxford

FENWICK A L
Oxford

FINE J H
London

FISHER M W
Ruthin

FLEMING F W
Glasgow

FLETCHER R
Prudhoe

FORD M
London

FORTH C E
Worcester Park

GABARRA A G
Kings Langley

GAMA R M
Guildford

GARDINER B M
London

GATENBY S J
London

GEORGE N V
Rugby

GILLESPIE M
Oxshott

GILMORE K
London

GLASER M
London

GODFREY J E
London

GOODALL J A D
Isle of Lewis

GREAVES E
Hitchin

GREENWOOD M C
London

GROUT J
Rochford

GUIRGUIS W R
Ipswich

GURR M I
Surrey

HALL J R
Basingstoke

HANSELL A
London

HARRISON J E
London

HIMAYAKANTHAN S
Maidstone

HOCHULI V K
Maidstone

HOLLOWAY B R
Macclesfield

HUGHES J M
London

HUGHES M C
Harlow

HUTTON J
Birmingham

ILES C A
London

JACKSON P G
London

JACKSON R A
London

JENKINS J C
Cirencester

JILANI M M
Abergavenny

KENNERLEY H
Oxford

KOSCHINSKA M
Wrexham

KYNASTON C
Llangollen

LEIGH F S M
Bath

LEONARD M
London

LEWIS D
Leigh

LEWIS J P
Barnet

LONG G
Portsmouth

MACKAY I
London

MARKS J
Cambridge

MARSDEN A P
Gloucester

MATHEW H
Dewsbury

McCRORY K
Nuneaton

McKENNA
Newcastle

MIDDLETON S J
High Wycombe

MILNER-SMITH S
Norwich

MILTON J E
London

MOORE D
Basingstoke

MORRIS J
London

MORTIMER R
Norwich

MUIR A
Basingstoke

MYERS J L
London

OHANIAN
Isleworth

O'HARA MAY A J
Brighton

O'KANE M
Leeds

OLLERENSHAW P L
Sidcup

OSWICK C M
Barnstaple

PALMER V V
Harrow

PAWAN G L S
London

PEVELER R C
Oxford

PHILLIPS G
Belfast

PORTEOUS J R
Oxford

POSTLE M K
Basingstoke

PRICE P A
Swindon

PRIOR T
Norwich

RAO B S
Macclesfield

RATH E A
London

REEVE E
Weybridge

RICHARDSON P C
Bishop Stortford

RIDDLE A J
London

ROBBINS L
Norwich

ROBINSON C H
London

ROBINSON J M
Langford

RODIE P
Redbridge

ROLLAND Y R
Slough

ROSE H
Quorn

ROY S
Wickford

SALEH F
Dorset

SALMONS P H
Dudley

SALTER C M
Brighton

SALVATONI A
Italy

SAMUEL G
Basingstoke

SANDERS M
London

SCHER Y M C
Southend-on-Sea

SCHILLER J
Pinner

SEYMOUR D P
London

SHAMMUGADASON S
Stevenage

SIMKINS M J
Epsom

SIMONS P J
Rochester

SINNETT L
London

SPALDING E
Birmingham

STEEL G
Bury St Edmunds

STEPHENSON P
Gateshead

STUTTAFORD I T
London

SUMMERBELL C
London

SUMMERS H
London

SUTTON C
Thornton Heath

TANG O T
Sheffield

THOMPSON R L
Harrow

THORPE D
Wokingham

THURGOOD S
Romsey

TODD J W
Farnham

VATERLAWS A L
Llandudno

WATT K A
Kettering

WEBBER S
Hingham

WELCH A A
Horley

WELCH K
St Albans

WHALEBELLY D
Colchester

WHITEHOUSE A M
Cambridge

WIDGINGTON N J
High Wycombe

WIGHTON J A
Buckingham

WILSON A L
London

WILSON A M
Cirencester